Maternal Health in India

Maternal Health in India

Contemporary Issues and Challenges

Edited by

Mohammad Akram

RAWAT PUBLICATIONS
Jaipur • New Delhi • Bangalore • Hyderabad • Guwahati • Kolkata

ISBN 978-81-316-0652-0

Published by
Prem Rawat for **Rawat Publications**
Satyam Apartments, Sector 3, Jawahar Nagar, Jaipur 302 004 (India)
Phone: 0141 265 1748/7006; Fax: 0141 265 1748
E-mail: info@rawatbooks.com
Website: www.rawatbooks.com

New Delhi Office
4858/24, Ansari Road, Daryaganj, New Delhi 110 002
Phone: 011 2326 3290

Also at *Bangalore, Hyderabad, Guwahati* and *Kolkata*

Typeset by
Mukesh Technologies Pvt. Ltd. Puducherry

Printed at
Nice Printing Press, New Delhi

Contents

Part II
Reproductive Trajectory: From Pregnancy to Childbirth

Part III
Diversities and Deprivations: Maternal Health Contextualized

Contributors

Mohammad Akram, Department of Sociology, Aligarh Muslim University, Aligarh.

Madhu Nagla, Department of Sociology, M.D. University, Rohtak.

K.R. Nayar, Santhigiri Social Research Institute, Trivandrum.

Lekha Bhat, Department of Social Work, Mizoram Central University, Aizwal.

Suchitra Pradhan, Odisha Watershed Development Mission, Siripur, Bhubaneswar.

Suhita Chopra Chatterjee, Department of Humanities and Social, Sciences, Indian Institute of Technology, Kharagpur.

Afzal Sayeed, Department of Social Work, Aligarh Muslim University, Aligarh.

Sayantika Palit, Centre for the Study of Social Systems, School of Social Sciences (CSSS/SSS), Jawaharlal Nehru University, New Delhi.

Mohd. Shahid, Aligarh Muslim University, Department of Social Work, Maulana Azad National Urdu University (MANUU), Hyderabad.

Anil Hiwale, Bhusawal Arts, Science and P.O., Nahata Commerce College, Bhusawal.

Ajay Choudhary, Department of Sociology, Hislop College, Nagpur.

Thounaojam Sunitibala Devi, Department of Sociology, Aligarh Muslim University, Aligarh.

Shakuntala C. Shettar, Professor, Department of Sociology, Karnatak University, Dharwad.

Nida Siddiqui, Department of Social Work, Aligarh Muslim University, Aligarh.

Rajiya Shahani, Department of Sociology, Assam University, Silchar.

Sylvia Fernandez Rao, National Institute of Nutrition (Indian Council of Medical Research), Hyderabad.

N. Balakrishna, National Institute of Nutrition (Indian Council of Medical Research), Hyderabad.

Patrice L. Engle, Department of Psychology and Child Development, Cal Poly State University, San Luis Obispo, CA.

Margaret (Peggy) Bentley, Institute for Global Health & Infectious Diseases. UNC Gillings School of Global Public Health, Chapel Hill, North Carolina.

Shahnaz Vazir, National Institute of Nutrition (Indian Council of Medical Research), Hyderabad.

M. Thamilarasan, Department of Sociology, University of Madras, Chennai.

M. Suganya, Department of Sociology, University of Madras, Chennai.

Introduction

This edited volume is an effort to locate the various contemporary issues related to maternal health in India and present multifaceted analysis from different perspectives. It presents empirical and analytical studies conducted in India mainly from 'social determinants of health' approach. It includes studies conducted in different parts of the country. The studies cover the underperforming states as well as the better-performing states. The papers address issues related to maternal health in the states of Uttar Pradesh, Madhya Pradesh, Andhra Pradesh, Odisha, Haryana, Manipur, Karnataka, Tamil Nadu and Kerala. A wide range of methods have been used by the contributors, including quantitative and qualitative methods. It includes papers on women's health, maternal health care, health status of pregnant women, antenatal care and delivery practices, needs of adolescent girls, health of rural women, maternal health policies and impact of Accredited Social Health Activist (ASHA), etc. It also includes non-conventional topics such as ethics and rights, technology and pain management, etc., which are pioneer studies and have not been studied at length before. The papers are thematically organized under three sections: 'maternal health: concepts and dimensions'; 'reproductive trajectory: from pregnancy to childbirth'; and 'diversities and deprivations: maternal health contextualized'.

Fourteen papers included in the volume share a common theme of exploring the social causation of differential experiences in maternal health. The varying and often unequal outcomes in maternal health have wider implications for the development trajectories and harmonious functioning of the nation state. The inequality in maternal health has strong relationship with infant mortality and child health. The maternal and child health (MCH) are intrinsically related to overall health structure. In a country such as India, which is characterized by multiple deprivations based on caste, class, gender and spatial distribution, inequalities in health outcomes have a much pervading impact. The sociocultural and politico-administrative barriers restrict the optimum utilization of whatever little health care facilities are available. The scanty presence of public health facilities, in many of the states, weakens the impact of the clinical interventions. Medical managerialism, ad hoc targetism and incoherent policy-making diminishes the enabling capacity of health. Unavailability of basic health goods, such as nutritious food, potable water and basic sanitation, for majority of the population reduces the chances of remaining healthy. The privatization of health care facilities and consequent increasing health expenditure is causing large-scale pauperization. Hence, it is important to locate the issues related to maternal health within the larger prevailing health structures and policies in India.

The unequal outcomes of health among various social categories are raising serious doubts about universal applicability of 'biomedical determinants of health approach' in the contemporary world. The 'social determinants of health approach' (which includes class, gender, ethnicity, education and occupation as determinants of health) along with 'political economics' of availability, accessibility and affordability of health environment and health care facilities are providing the much needed explanations of the causation of trajectories of hiatus and inequities in health outcomes of various social and spatial categories. Judicious distribution of basic amenities and promotion of health care facilities, both governmental and non-governmental, is suggested as the dominant 'remedial' as well as 'facilitating' paradigm for mitigating the health inequities and achieving the goals of 'health for all'. The wide gaps even in the outcomes of health care facilities, as reflected through indicators such as life expectancy at birth, maternal mortality, infant mortality, morbidity patterns, etc., despite claims of 'reforms', 'revamps' and 'realignments' in policies, plans and programmes, raise serious questions not only about effective implementation of the development programmes but also about 'acceptability' and 'administration' of the health care efforts.

Acceptability is normally considered a cultural issue and comes into focus whenever 'corrections', 'innovations', 'adoptions' and 'transformations' are introduced. Acceptance of technology-induced health-related interventions such as test-tube baby, surrogacy, hired womb, sex-change, organ transplantation, etc., depends on cultural patterns as well as several other socio-economic factors. However, acceptance of medicine or other health care provisions as a means of treatment for disease or ill health depends on complex discourses and interplays among and between the macro-level structures and the micro-level perceptions. Administration is another important factor that decides not only the quality of implementation of various intervention programmes at various levels, but also the degree or level of engagement/disengagement such interventions may generate. Poor or maladministration leads to poor acceptance of such paradigms and causes marginalization of several social categories in those contexts. Hence, any effort to understand the differential outcomes of institutional health care (e.g. institutional delivery, family planning, vaccination or immunization) among various social and spatial categories in India needs to take into consideration the cultural ethos of acceptability and the contested formalism of administrative mechanisms also.

The Preamble to the World Health Organization Constitution affirms that it is one of the fundamental rights of every human being to enjoy the highest attainable standards of health. The Universal Declaration of Human Rights mentions in Article 25 that everyone has the right to a standard of living adequate for the health and well-being of himself and his family. Similarly, Article 21 of the Constitution of India guarantees 'right to life' to its citizens and health is an integral aspect of human life. Thus, health is human being's birth right. Improving health status of the citizens is one of the most important goals of all the modern welfare governments. Health status of a population and especially of the vulnerable population such as women, children, indigenous population, unorganized workers, etc., is considered as an important indicator of development. Health is increasingly being seen as a development issue rather than just a medical issue. Ill health and poor access to health services are seen as indicators of poor economics, irresponsible policy-making and immoral politics.

The Alma Ata Declaration of 1978 stated that attainment of the highest possible level of health is the most important worldwide social goal and its realization requires the action of many other social and economic sectors in addition to the health sector. It also says that the existing gross inequality in the health status of the people, particularly between developed and developing countries, as well as within countries, is politically, socially and economically unacceptable and is, therefore, of common concern to all countries. The declaration made its vision very clear: health for all the people of the world by the year 2000. However, the goal of health for all remained an illusion in various parts of the developing world including India till the end of the last century. Responding to the unmet health needs even after two decades of the Alma Ata Declaration and coming into existence of other health complications, the world had the Millennium Development Goals (MDGs) at the turn of the century, specifying the various development targets (including health-related targets) to be achieved in the early decades of the twenty-first century.

The Alma Ata Declaration and many other studies carried out in the last two decades of the twentieth century exposed the widespread inequalities inherent in the health condition of the people. The inequalities in health are not simply the indicators of the inequalities present in various other segments of the society, but they do have their own 'independent existence' because of the presence of several sociocultural and politico-administrative marginalization and even exclusion processes. Health inequality, according to Amartya Sen, is one of the basic forms of inequality. Health inequality does not mean just some kind of health difference, but the differences in health, which adversely affect the opportunities and performances of those afflicted by it and are potentially avoidable through policy correction. Health inequality is often expressed as health inequity. It is a difference in which disadvantaged social groups (such as poor, indigenous population, racial/ethnic minorities, women, children, unorganized workers and other groups that have persistently experienced social disadvantage or discrimination) systematically experience worse health or greater health risks than more advantaged social groups.

Cross-national evidences suggest that greater the degree of socio-economic inequality that exist within a society, the steeper the gradient of health inequality. Studies reveal that middle-income groups in a more unequal society have worse health than comparable or even poorer groups in a society with greater equality. However, health inequality is not always the result of economic inequality. The differences in health among individuals in society are different from inequalities between social groups. Health inequality refers to the group inequalities and not individual differences within the groups. Contemporary literature from noble laureates suggest that inequalities in health often have much more negative consequences than the income inequalities as health has both instrumental and intrinsic value, whereas income has only instrumental value. Inequalities in health cause deprivation as they adversely affect the capability of people to function.

India has witnessed more than six decades of planned intervention in combating diseases and promoting health care since its independence. Health is a state subject in the Indian Constitution, though the Centre plays an important role as a regulator, advisor and resource provider. The government is obligated to provide health care to every citizen of India without any discrimination on the basis of creed, colour, race, sex and place of residence. India had its first National Health Policy (NHP) in 1983. The second NHP came in 2002. The National Rural Health Mission (NRHM) was launched in 2005 to ensure participation of the local self-government institutions at village and panchayat levels in a meaningful way. Although policies come into existence and operate within political systems, they get guided not only by the state actors or societal needs but also by the processes and mechanisms through which they come into existence and operate. Health policy needs to be understood by taking into consideration the discourses, processes and power relations. It involves exploring the role of the state, the actors at the national and international levels, the external (corporate and interest groups) forces influencing it and the mechanism within the political system for participation in policy making. States are not always the sovereign decision makers, especially in the economic sphere. Hence, it is also important to take into consideration the important milestones in the development of health policy in general, and programmes and planning related to maternal health in particular, while understanding the coming into existence of maternal health policies.

With this background, the papers included in the volume elaborately analyse the different dimensions of maternal health in India. Mohammad Akram defines various conceptual issues and presents an overview of maternal health in India. Maternal health refers to the health of women during pregnancy, childbirth and the postpartum period. Throughout human history, pregnancy and childbearing have caused death and disability both among women and neonatal.

Pregnancy and childbirth are of course not diseases. But they carry risks because of the varying and embedded complications, practices, processes, beliefs, life conditions and the immediate environment. These risks can be reduced by health care interventions such as the provision of maternal and public health care, supplementary nutrition, family planning, safe abortion and improvement in other reproductive conditions. Taking an overview of the health care patterns and structures in India and relying on data provided by National Family Health Survey (NFHS), Sample Registration System, Millennium Development Goals-India Country Report (MDG-ICR) and other sources, Akram tries to locate the achievements and underachievements in maternal health in India. The paper tries to address the scope of primary health care and public health priorities within the context and also suggests measures for improvement.

Madhu Nagla examines the historical and contemporary ethical concerns on women in medicine. Her paper summarizes major principles around which much of ethics debates concerning medical and health care have been organized. Her paper connects the medical ethics in India with the contemporary concern. The paper is divided into two parts: The first part attempts to discuss historical development of medical ethics at a global level and the second part attempts to discuss the historical aspects of medical ethics in India. According to Nagla, western philosophy has been profoundly shaped by three theories of ethics: Aristotelianism, deontology and utilitarianism. Each of these three theories can in turn be seen as essentially a product of the times in which it was originally born. The discourses of ethics and moral conclude that they are inseparable from local relations and conditions and at the same time aspire for trans-local perspective. Importantly, the four principles of ethics, that is, autonomy, beneficence, non-maleficence and justice are prima facie and binding for each individual to follow.

Medical ethics are not merely a moral code but a legally sanctioned code of conduct that is acceptable and normal within the medical profession. A broad range of issues can be covered under the rubric of ethical issues; however, specific concerns related to the globalization, equity in health, technology and ethics, informed consent, emergency and health care and reproduction are the major concern of ethics. The ideas enshrined in the doctrine of informed consent, although not legally binding, continue to percolate into the medical and lay discourse. The doctrine of informed consent is complicated and needs to be addressed in sociocultural and other constraints of the society. Advances in biosciences and biotechnology, such as surrogacy, sex selection, genetics, etc., widened the scope of medical ethics. Ethics are the bridge between health policy and values. Health policy is related with the equity and justice to the people in receiving health care, and thus medical ethics examines the moral validity of it. Nagla feels that there is a need to develop an ethical culture in society. Ethics, equity and respect for humanity must be incorporated in all aspects of health care. Ethics has to be institutionalized wherever it is needed. Given the events of the past decades, it is a sad reality that at least in the Indian health care set-up, ethics are losing their sight and has been moving towards commercialization than in science and healing.

K.R. Nayar and Lekha Bhat examine the social determinants of Mother and Child Health (MCH) in India from macro–micro disjunction perspective. According to them, the central issues with respect to maternity care from a sociological viewpoint are social exclusion and inequalities and the issue of social dignity when the women utilize institutions for birthing. Their paper examines social dimensions such as social exclusion and dignity with respect to maternal health and maternal health care using macro and micro data and demonstrates the disjunctions with macro and micro data with respect to outcomes of the programmes initiated in recent times. Macro data from several states indicate quantitative increase in the utilization of institutional care from which one can assume that issues of exclusion and marginalization have narrowed. However, it is necessary to examine whether such quantitative increase has led to well-being of women who seek care especially in terms of actual reductions in exclusion and improvements in terms of dignity of birthing. This is attempted in this paper through an inductive process attempted in two public hospitals as part of a larger study to understand the processes and the context in which human dignity is violated in maternity wards of public hospitals in Kerala.

Nayar and Bhat find that the disjunction between macro and micro realities, which is evident from the data, is important from both a methodological and programme point of view. Methodologically, it shows the need for triangulation while reaching conclusions on programme effectiveness. The disjunctions between macro and micro data and deduction and induction could be explored further by undertaking studies in other states. Increasing institutional deliveries using conditional cash transfers or using other incentives through the Janani Suraksha Yojana (JSY) are important from the programme point of view. The sudden off-take of maternity services in vulnerable states leads us to assume that the social questions such as exclusion and marginalization have been addressed or the gap is narrowing. However, micro data from the state of Kerala, which is one of the better-performing states of India, show the contrary picture. The empirical observations demonstrate the vulnerabilities of women when they reach the institutions for birthing. The indignities they go through and the exclusion and marginalization they face are the negative lessons worth considering for improving the maternal health programmes.

Suchitra Pradhan and Suhita Chopra Chatterjee, in their paper on assessing the benefits of cancer screening programmes in Odisha, methodologically examine the truth and relevance of the argument that regular use of screening methods can detect cancers of the breast, colon, rectum, cervix and prostate at an early stage, in the Indian context. National Cancer Programmes worldwide rely heavily on screening for early detection of breast and cervical cancer. However, in recent times, there have been polarized arguments about the benefits and harm of screening. Their paper looks into some of the ethical debates and questions the value of screening in India. Based on a study in Odisha, they identify the structural and socio-economic barriers, which make screening programmes lose their efficacy in India. In the light of the arguments presented, their paper asks for a serious scientific rethinking of screening measures to save financial costs and redirect resources for evolving better treatment modalities.

Afzal Sayeed in his paper contextualizes MCH policies and planning in India since the colonial era. For Sayeed, health and well-being of the citizen is the most valuable asset for any country, and their care is the most sacred commitment of any government. The development of any society can be measured by the quality of health care delivery services in general and MCH care in particular. India is an age-old civilization. This long history is also marked by a shadow of imperial rule for about two centuries. The colonial era was marked by more individual voluntary efforts that lacked organized planning pertaining to MCH. India, on attaining independence, embarked upon the 'socialist pattern' of planned development. This paper is an attempt to go into the annals of historical development in the realm of Mother and Child Health (MCH) situations, policy, programme and outcomes. Based on secondary sources such as various reports, policy documents, plan papers and specific programmes, this paper explores the roots of present policies and programmes and focuses on the evolution of health planning in general and MCH in particular. The paper finds that even after decades of planning and programme implementation, India remains one of the unhealthiest countries of the world; painting unimpressive pictures in respect of all health indicators and MCH services are no exception. The paper suggests that we need to restructure the overall policies and programmes for achieving a healthy society.

Sayantika Palit, in her paper on a sociological analysis of pain during childbirth, states that pain is perceived as being intrinsic to childbirth. One of the first principles of treatment in modern medicine is that when pain is present, it should be relieved as soon as possible. However, in some cultures, pain is seen as so central to childbirth that without it no childbirth is seen to be possible, and any effort towards its relief is considered against the will of nature. Thus, childbirth and pain management is a complex subject and has many historical layers to it. It is as much a physiological process as it is a cultural phenomenon. It is not simply about what is best for the mother and child, but it involves a host of sociocultural factors. This paper explores the different facets to this subject and also looks at the different debates that surround the issue of pain management in childbirth.

Various forms of technology are involved in the management of pain with different degrees of success and acceptance among labouring women. There was a period in America and Europe when pain relief through medical intervention was sought as a right that every woman should have. Today, there is again a resurgence of the homebirth movement where some women want to embrace the pain of labour and experience childbirth. But, it is also true that the rates of C-section have gone up in most developed and developing economies as it is seen as the best means to reduce 'risks' associated with childbirth and also ensure that pain is minimal. The biomedical model of birth dismissed natural births attended to by family and midwives as unscientific and risky. It assumed that maternal mortality and morbidity can be lowered only by use of technology. But it is important to go a little deeper and investigate before accepting such claims, which is what the paper of Sayantika Palit makes an endeavour to do.

Mohd. Shahid in his paper on reproductive repertoire states that marriage, pregnancy and childbirth constitute important markers of rites of passage across societies. In India, there are culturally approved notions, rites and rituals denoting prescriptions and proscriptions, celebration or no celebration on the events relating to marriage and fertility in general, and pregnancy and childbirth, in particular. These constitute collective memory, and narratives around these may vary across cultures; but in each culture, these are passed on from generation to generation. How do people make sense of the marriage and fertility issues and to what extent sociocultural context guides and governs the popular perception? Is the popular common sense on issues of marriage and fertility, in general, and pregnancy and childbirth, in particular, hegemonic in nature? Does it represent dominant constructions and legitimize biasness and prejudices for the other – they may be women (gender-based discrimination), rural population (region-specific stereotypes), minorities (religion-centric prejudices) and many more such groups on the other side of the power spectrum? Shahid's paper focuses on some such questions and endeavours to interrogate how popular common sense upholds and sustains the hegemonic constructions on the issues of marriage and fertility. Using Gramsci's notion of common sense, Shahid attempts to understand the reproductive repertoire and the subterranean linkages around gender, region and religion. The discussion on reproductive repertoire with Gramscian gaze helps to locate the biases, blames and stereotyping across gender, region and religion, which are the rampant and running themes on the issues of reproductive health.

Anil Hiwale and Ajay Choudhary consider health as a basic human right for all individuals. Inequalities in health are pervasive within states and among social groups in India. Even in states, where aggregate health indicators are improving, some health gaps between population groups are widening or remaining stagnant. Despite the government efforts to reach out to pregnant women in all parts of the country to provide all components of maternal health care free or with nominal charges, utilization of maternal health remains low in the country. The study focuses on the maternal health utilization by residence, educational level and wealth index among social groups in Madhya Pradesh, where the infant mortality rate is the third highest among the states of India. The data used for the study come from the National Family

Health Survey-3 conducted in 2005–06 (NFHS-3). The results indicate that the factors such as residence, education, wealth index, etc., are statistically significant and affect the utilization of maternal health care among social groups in Madhya Pradesh. The findings of the study are used to provide insights for the creation of more efficient and beneficial planning of maternal health service delivery.

Thounaojam Sunitibala Devi in her paper examines the reproductive health and developmental needs of adolescent girls in Manipur. Adolescence is usually a time of good health for girls but also a time of risk, particularly regarding their lack of awareness on their health care, reproductive health, sexual activity and substance use. Preventing and dealing with such risks is necessary for their health, as adolescents account for the initial period of the reproductive age group. The health of adolescents sets the stage for their future health and well-being, as well as for the health of their children and the development of the society as well. The paper finds that due to lack of awareness, adolescent girls in Manipur suffer from mental stress and face problems because of the physiological, psychological and social changes that have taken place due to the onset of puberty. They also lack information on hygiene practices during menstruation, which may consequently increase susceptibility to various infections. The result shows that adolescent girls are inadequately addressed and are a more vulnerable group. There is a need to create awareness among adolescent girls so that they enjoy good health in the society.

For Shakuntala C. Shettar, maternal health is a critical topic in health care. Maternal illness, health and death impact families, communities and societies and have far-reaching effect across socio-economic strata. Despite recent data showing a positive turning point in the battle to keep mothers alive through pregnancy care and childbirth support, the maternal mortality rate is still high in India, and significant gender-based health disparities remain perpetuated. Limited access to education and employment, high illiteracy and increasing poverty level is making health improvements for women exceedingly difficult. Shettar's paper is an effort to understand the barriers in maternal health and care in rural India. Her paper concludes that national government, non-government organizations and other important players must commit to address policy barriers for improving maternal health, including efforts to increasing resources for health care systems.

According to Nida Siddiqui, millions of people in developing countries are trapped in poverty, malnutrition, hunger and disease. There are regional variations in terms of prevailing living conditions among various spatial categories, and the rural sections of the society are the most vulnerable because of very limited access to resources. The resources are generally short: the World Health Organization has identified a global deficit of nearly 4.3 million health workers. The use of para-professional health workers has been provisioned in several countries to close the health worker gap. Although community health workers cannot replace a weak health system, they can perform valuable tasks such as case management for common illnesses, promotion of desired health behaviour, immunization and awareness generation. Siddiqui looks at the latest band of community-based functionaries, named ASHA, which was proposed under NRHM to serve the population of 1,000 in hilly areas and 500 in desert terrain in rural areas. ASHA is the first port of call for any health-related demands of deprived sections of the population, especially women, children, aged, sick and disabled people. She is the link between the community and the health care provider. Siddiqui's paper tries to find out the impact of ASHA on maternal as well as child health. It finds that age and level of education of ASHA affected the diet of pregnant women, household visits and health checkups during pregnancy and first visit of ASHA after the delivery. A higher educational level of ASHA was related to better performance in all parameters except household visit made by ASHA. Hence, appointment of trained and qualified ASHA can give the much desired impetus to the weakly constructed maternal health care efforts.

According to Rajiya Shahani, antenatal care and delivery health practices have been the central themes in the agenda of today's welfare-oriented women's reproductive health programmes. The emergence of safe motherhood is a priority area of MCH care programmes, so that all women receive the care they need to be safe and healthy through pregnancy and childbirth. The notion of safe motherhood refers to a strategy of reducing the maternal mortality and morbidity through the promotion of skilled birth attendants and delivery in hygienic environment. This is mainly due to the fact that most maternal deaths occur close to time of delivery and that the major causes of maternal death require medical interventions. Maternal health requires urgent attention, as there is an extraordinary difference in maternal death rates between the developed and developing countries. According to the World Bank, about one-third of the total disease burden of women of 15–44 years of age in developing countries is linked to health problems related to pregnancy. Every time a woman in the Third World becomes pregnant, her risk of dying is 200 times higher than the risk run by a woman in the developed world. In many developing countries about 50 per cent of pregnancy terminations occur among the high-risk mothers. The magnitude of such women's reproductive health problems still remains immense.

Shahani conducted her study among the married Muslim women of Yangbi Khoonou village in Imphal East district, Manipur and finds that the unawareness is the major factor that deprives the respondents from using the proper antenatal care and scientific health care practices. The mothers who do not seek the proper antenatal care practices are mostly uneducated. Apart from the illiteracy and unawareness, there are some other factors that act as barriers in using modern practices of antenatal health, some of these are distance from the health services centre, feeling not necessary, inconvenience to accept or avail facilities, no botheration shown by the husband, elders health staff, etc.

Sylvia Fernandez Rao, N. Balakrishna, Patrice L. Engle, Margaret (Peggy) Bentley and Shahnaz Vazir study the role of maternal locus of control causing behaviour change in infant and young child feeding interventions within rural communities. In this study, a randomized controlled trial was carried out for a year among rural mothers in Andhra Pradesh, India. Six hundred mothers and infants (three months old) were selected. There were two intervention groups and a control group. The intervention included nutrition education on breast feeding and complementary feeding by a trained village worker (Group 2) and education on responsive feeding, child development stimulation and nutrition education for one group (Group 3). Group 1 served as the control. Maternal locus of control and child growth and development were assessed after 12 months of intervention.

Maternal locus of control (LOC) scores significantly differed ($p < 0.05$) according to level of maternal education. Higher education showed (8.3) a stronger internal orientation. Children of mothers with external LOC in Group 2 had lesser growth faltering (significance $p = 0.08$) compared to the children in the internal LOC category of both the control and Group 3. The mean mental and motor index scores according to the maternal LOC showed no difference among internals of both intervention groups. Externals who received the intervention also had a mean score (106) similar to the internals. These results show that an internal maternal locus of control is beneficial for the mental development of the child and externals benefit more from education interventions in rural communities.

M. Thamilarasan and M. Suganya in their study based on descriptive design attempt to analyse the health condition of pregnant women belonging to Scheduled Caste. The paper studies the changes that are occurring during pregnancy and the level of awareness the respondents possess about their own health condition during pregnancy. The paper finds that 70 per cent of the respondents (pregnant women) are aware of their health condition and the value of nutritional food and had started to concentrate on their health and hygiene. Most among the remaining, though aware of their health condition, are not in a position to take any specific efforts for improvement due to poverty, illiteracy, low income and so on. A pregnant woman has emotional feelings after the confirmation of her pregnancy. Majority of the respondents (pregnant women) feel happy about their pregnancy. However, 2 per cent of respondents wished to abort the pregnancy due to several reasons. The findings suggest that the large portion of the pregnant women get all kind of support from their family members. Further, the pregnant women perceive that working during the pregnancy is good exercise and helps in easy delivery of the child. The paper concludes that quality health care, offering information and counselling, enables women to make informed decisions about their health.

Thus, this volume aims at exploring the social causation of poor maternal health in India. The book includes papers related to several interrelated sub-themes such as social determinants of maternal health in India; political economics of proper health care for women; availability, accessibility, affordability and acceptability of institutional health care facilities; evaluation of maternal health programmes and policies; and, deprivations, marginalization and exclusions related to maternal health. The core theme of the volume is to address the diversities, differential achievements and challenges in maternal health in contemporary India amidst the well claimed wide range reforms and periodic compounding of various health programmes. It is important to note here that there are several global-and national-level reports on maternal health emphasizing more on government programmes than presenting evaluation of such programmes or assessment of ground realities. The micro-level nuances based on objective and scientific research analysis is missing in them. There are studies on reproductive health issues also, but they hardly include the comprehensive parameters and indicators related to maternal health. While fulfilling the need of quest for knowledge for the inquisitive minds and the need of scientific and meticulous information for the policy makers and administrators, this volume intends to provide the much needed theoretically informed and methodologically sound comprehensive papers and fill up the identified gaps.

Mohammad Akram

Part I

Maternal Health: Concepts and Dimensions

CHAPTER 1

Maternal Health in India: An Overview

Mohammad Akram

Maternal health is a key indicator of women's health and status. Maternal health refers to the health of women during pregnancy, childbirth and the postpartum period. Although motherhood is often a positive and fulfilling experience, for many women, it is associated with suffering, ill health and even death. Throughout human history, pregnancy and childbearing have caused death and disability in both women and neonates. Pregnancy and childbirth are of course not diseases (WHO, 2009). But, they carry risks because of the varying and embedded complications, practices, processes, beliefs, life conditions and the immediate environment. These risks can be reduced by health care interventions such as the provision of maternal and public health care, supplementary nutrition, family planning, safe abortion and improvement in other reproductive conditions. Maternal death may be caused by the interplay of several interlinked factors: medical conditions directly associated with childbearing (e.g. haemorrhage, sepsis, eclampsia, obstructed labour); other health and disease conditions (e.g. malaria, heart disease, other communicable and non-communicable diseases); and socio-economic factors such as patterns of gender politics that result in early marriage and high fertility, and compromise of access to nutrition, health care and contraception, especially amongst the poor, villagers and marginalized communities (Jeffery and Jeffery, 2010).

Reducing maternal death and morbidity has been a major focus for the developing world since the launch of the Safe Motherhood Initiative in 1987 (WHO, 1996). Millennium Development Goals

(MDGs), at the turn of the century, gave a further impetus to the goals of making the world safe for both the mothers and the newborn. Evidence suggests that the sociocultural determinants of maternal, newborn and child health have a cumulative effect over a lifetime. A correlation exists between the social inequity and maternal and child health (WHO, 2005). In industrialized countries, there are on an average 9 maternal deaths per 100,000 live births, whereas in the most disadvantaged countries, this figure can be as high as 1,000 or more per 100,000 live births (WHO, 2009). India, in recent past, is witnessing a gradual decline in both maternal and neonatal mortalities because of several planned interventions. But such decline is not uniform among various social and spatial categories. Further, decline in maternal mortality cannot be taken as the absolute indicator of sound maternal health as reproductive concerns and overall health conditions of women have important bearing upon maternal health. Within the framework of World Health Organization (WHO)'s definition of health as a state of complete physical, mental and social well-being, and not merely the absence of disease or infirmity, reproductive health addresses the reproductive processes, functions and systems at all stages of life (WHO, 2006).

The Universal Declaration of Human Rights (1948) stated in Article 25: 'Everyone has the right to a standard of living adequate for the health and wellbeing of himself and his family...' (United Nations, 1948). The WHO was established in 1948 with the objective of attaining the highest possible level of health for all people. Right to life, as stated in Article 21 of the Constitution of India, does not only mean biological existence but also life of a dignified human being with all its concomitant attributes, which may include food to eat, potable water to drink, nutrition, life skill, education, healthy environment and effective health care facilities (Akram, 2007, 2012a). Within this broad framework, this paper intends to locate the state of maternal health in India after six decades of planned change and health interventions. Looking beyond the germ theory that emphasizes only on the biomedical determinants of health, this paper tries to take a comprehensive approach by including the sociocultural, the politico-administrative and the macro-environmental determinants of maternal health. Taking an overview of the health care patterns and structures in India and relying on data provided by the National Family Health Survey (NFHS), Sample Registration System (SRS), MDG-India Country Report (MDG-ICR) and other authentic sources, the paper tries to locate the achievements and underachievements in maternal health in India. It also tries to address the scope of primary health care and public health priorities within the context and suggests measures for improvement.

MATERNAL DEATH: GLOBAL AND NATIONAL CONCERNS

In the international statistical classification of diseases and related health problems (ICD-10), WHO defines maternal death as the death of a woman while pregnant or within 42 days of termination of pregnancy, irrespective of the duration and the site of the pregnancy, from any cause related to or aggravated by the pregnancy or its management, but not from accidental or incidental causes. It further states that a late maternal death is the death of a woman from direct or indirect obstetric causes for more than 42 days but less than 1 year after termination of pregnancy (WHO, 2011: 156). Maternal deaths, according to this classification, should be subdivided into two groups: direct obstetric deaths—which are those resulting from obstetric complications of the pregnant state (pregnancy, labour and puerperium), from interventions, omissions, incorrect treatment or a chain of events resulting from any of the above; and indirect obstetric deaths—which are those resulting from previous existing disease or disease that developed during pregnancy and which was not due to direct obstetric causes, but which was aggravated by physiological effects of pregnancy.

The latest estimates issued by the WHO, the United Nations Population Fund (UNFPA), the United Nations Children's Fund (UNICEF) and the World Bank (WB) in September 2010 provide figures related to maternal death: globally, an estimated 287,000 maternal deaths occurred in 2010. Sub-Saharan Africa (56 per cent) and Southern Asia (29 per cent) accounted for 85 per cent of the global burden in 2010. At the country level, two countries account for one-third of global maternal deaths: India at 19 per cent and Nigeria at 14 per cent. Maternal mortality ratio (MMR) measures the number of women aged 15–49 years dying due to maternal causes per 100,000 live births. The global MMR in 2010 was 210 maternal deaths per 100,000 live births. The MMR in developing regions (240) was 15 times higher than in developed regions. Sub-Saharan Africa had the highest MMR at 500 maternal deaths per 100,000 live births. The MMRs of the remaining developing regions, in descending order of maternal deaths per 100,000 live births, are Southern Asia (220), Oceania (200), South-eastern Asia (150), Latin America and the

Caribbean (80), Northern Africa (78), Western Asia (71), the Caucasus and Central Asia (46) and Eastern Asia (37) (WHO, 2012: 1).

The MMR in India is 212 per 100,000 live births according to SRS report for 2007–09 (SRS, 2011). There is a decline from the earlier ratio of 254 during 2004–06. Wide disparities exist across states in India. The MMR ranges from 81 in Kerala to 390 in Assam (during 2007–09) (see Table 1.1).

Table 1.1 Maternal Mortality Ratio (MMR); India, EAG* and Assam, Southern States and Other States, 2004–06 and 2007–09

India and Major States	*MMR 2004–06*	*MMR 2007–09*
INDIA TOTAL	254	212
Assam	480	390
Bihar/Jharkhand	312	261
Madhya Pradesh/Chhattisgarh	335	269
Odisha	303	258
Rajasthan	388	318
Uttar Pradesh/Uttarakhand	440	359
EAG AND ASSAM SUBTOTAL	375	308
Andhra Pradesh	154	134
Karnataka	213	178
Kerala	95	81
Tamil Nadu	111	97
SOUTH SUBTOTAL	149	127
Gujarat	160	148
Haryana	186	153
Maharashtra	130	104
Punjab	192	172
West Bengal	141	145
Other	206	160
OTHER SUBTOTAL	174	149

*Empowered Action Group (EAG).

Source: (SRS, 2011).

MDGs AND MATERNAL AND CHILD HEALTH: THE JOURNEY SO FAR

MDGs are the specific goals of social transformation designed for the entire world at the beginning of the twenty-first century. MDGs are a set of numerical and time-bound targets to measure achievements in human and social development. The MDGs originated from the Millennium Declaration produced by the United Nations. The Millennium Declaration outlined the most ambitious global agenda till date for eradicating poverty and preventable diseases, promoting equitable development and protecting the earth's environment. The Declaration asserted that every individual has the right to dignity, freedom, equality, a basic standard of living that includes freedom from hunger, disease and violence, and encourages tolerance and solidarity. The MDGs were made to operationalize these ideas by setting targets and indicators for poverty reduction and health improvement. The MDGs are eight international development goals that all 192 United Nations member states and at least 23 international organizations have agreed to achieve by the year 2015. The eight goals are to eradicate extreme poverty and hunger, achieve universal primary education; promote gender equality and empower women; reduce child mortality rates; improve maternal health, combat HIV/AIDS, malaria and other diseases; ensure environmental sustainability; and develop a global partnership for development. All these goals are directly or indirectly related to improvement in health status of individuals and communities. Major successes in combating extreme poverty, improving school enrolment and child health and controlling spread of killer diseases such as AIDS, malaria and tuberculosis in almost all developing countries—even in the poorest countries—demonstrate that the MDGs are achievable (MDG-ICR, 2011).

In India, women of reproductive age (15–45 years) and children (<15 years) constitute about 60 per cent of the total population. They comprise the vulnerable and less-empowered fraction of the population due to the risks connected with childbearing in case of women; and growth, development and survival in case of infants and children. Reduction of child mortality and improvement in maternal health are the major goals in the Millennium Declaration, to which India is a signatory. About one-fifth of the Indian population is in the adolescent age group and yet to begin their reproductive lives. It is expected that this age group will continue to grow. Thus, for all these

Table 1.2 Specific Maternal and Child Health Goals and Indicators of the MDGs

Goal No.	*Goals*	*Indicators*	*Targets by 2015*
4	Reduce infant mortality	Infant mortality rate (IMR)	28
	Reduce child mortality	Under 5 mortality rate (U5MR)	42
5	Improve maternal health	Maternal mortality ratio	109

Source: (SRS, 2011).

reasons, maternal, newborn and child health have become a priority area for the policy makers, planners and various professionals (WHO, 2005: 28) (Table 1.2).

As per SRS 2009, as reported by the MDG-ICR, 2011, the neonatal mortality rate (number of deaths of infants less than 29 days per thousand live births) for India was 34 (rural—38, urban—21). The infant mortality rate for the year 2009 consisting of neonatal and post-neonatal mortality cases for the country came down to 50 (rural—55, urban—34) with the percentage share of neonatal deaths to infant deaths 67.9 (rural—69.1, urban—61.0). SRS-based U5MR in India for the year 2009 stands at 64, and it varies from 71 in rural areas to 41 in urban areas. With a target to reduce U5MR to 42 per thousand live births by 2015, India tends to reach near to 54 per thousand live births by 2015, missing the target by 12 percentage points. The states that had U5MR above the national-level estimate (64) in 2009 are Madhya Pradesh (89), Assam (87), Uttar Pradesh (85), Odisha (84), Rajasthan (74), Bihar (70) and Chhattisgarh (67). Some of the states/union territories of the country have also shown a declining trend in U5MR. Kerala (14), Tamil Nadu (33), Maharashtra (36), Delhi (37) and West Bengal (40) have already achieved the all-India MDG target for 2015 with respect to U5MR. IMR in India has registered a 3-point decline to 50 in 2009 from 53 in 2008. The states of Madhya Pradesh (67), Odisha (65), Uttar Pradesh (63), Assam (61), Meghalaya (59), Rajasthan (59), Chhattisgarh (54), Bihar (52) and Haryana (51) reported IMR above the national estimates. It is important to note here that IMR of infant girls is consistently higher than IMR of infant boys in India, except in a few years over the past two decades. Uniformly over the years, a gap of three percentage points persists between IMR (male) and IMR (female).

Sample Registration System (SRS) data indicate that India has recorded a deep decline in MMR of 35 per cent from 327 during 1999–2001 to 212 during 2007–09 and a fall of about 17 per cent during 2006–09. The decline in MMR from 1990 to 2009 is 51 per cent. Among the age group of 15–49 years, 63 per cent of the maternal deaths were females in the age group of 20–29 years as per the 2007–09 SRS maternal mortality estimates. From an estimated MMR level of 437 per 100,000 live births during 1990–91, India is required to reduce the MMR to 109 per 100,000 live births by 2015. At this historical pace of decrease, India tends to reach MMR of 139 per 100,000 live births by 2015, falling short by 29 points. However, the bright line in the trend is the sharper decline, that is, 17 per cent during 2006–09 and 16 per cent during 2003–06 compared to 8 per cent decline during 2001–03. It is worth noting that the number of states that have adhered to the all-India MDG target during 2007–09 went up to 3 against 1, only till 2006. Kerala had the sole distinction of achieving the all-India MDG target for MMR in 2004–06. Tamil Nadu and Maharashtra are the new entrants. Andhra Pradesh, West Bengal, Gujarat and Haryana are in closer proximity to the all-India MDG target. Further, the states of Kerala, West Bengal, Bihar and Jharkhand are likely to achieve their state-level MMR targets by 2015, with the current trend continuing. However, from their 2007–09 levels, the states of Assam (390), Haryana (153) and Odisha (258) are likely to fall short of their state-level targets by huge margins. The remaining states are likely to miss the targets by 18–52 points (MDG-ICR, 2011).

HEALTH STRUCTURE AND PATTERNS

The health sector in India is characterized by (i) a government/public sector that provides publicly financed and managed curative and preventive health services from primary to tertiary level, throughout the country (these account for about 18 per cent of the overall health spending and 0.9 per cent of the GDP), and (ii) a fee-levying private sector that plays a dominant role in the provision of individual curative care through ambulatory services and accounts for about 82 per cent of the overall health expenditure and 4.2 per cent of the GDP. The provision of health care by the public sector is a responsibility shared by the state, central and local governments, although it is effectively a state responsibility in terms of service delivery. State and local governments incur about three-quarters and the centre about one-quarter of public spending on health. The responsibility for health is at three levels. First, health is primarily a state responsibility. Second, the centre is responsible for health services in union territories without a legislature and is also responsible for developing and monitoring national standards and regulations, linking the states with funding agencies and sponsoring numerous schemes for implementation by state governments. Third, both the centre and the states have a joint responsibility for programmes listed under the concurrent list. The goals and strategies for the public sector in health care are established through a consultative process involving all levels of government through the Central Council for Health and Family Welfare (Advani and Akram, 2007).

The organization of public sectors at the national level consists of the Union Ministry of Health and Family Welfare, which has three departments, namely Health, Family Welfare and Indian System of Medicine and Homeopathy. The organization at the state level is under the State Department of Health and Family Welfare in each state headed by a Minister and with a Secretariat under the charge of Secretary/Commissioner (Health and Family Welfare) belonging to the cadre of Indian Administrative Service. In the states of Bihar, Madhya Pradesh, Uttar Pradesh, Andhra Pradesh, Karnataka and others, zonal or regional or divisional set-ups have been created between the State Directorate of Health Services and District Health Administration. Each regional/zonal set-up covers three to five districts and acts under authority delegated by the State Directorate of Health Services. The district-level structure of health services is a middle-level management organization, and it is a link between the state as well as regional structure, on the one side, and the peripheral-level structures such as Primary Health Centres (PHCs) as well as sub-centre, on the other side. At the *taluka* level, health care services are rendered through the office of Assistant District Health and Family Welfare Officer. Some specialties are made available at the *taluka* hospital.

Further, one Community Health Centre has been established for every 80,000–120,000 population, and this centre provides the basic specialty services in general medicine, paediatrics, surgery, obstetrics and gynaecology. There is one PHC covering about 30,000 (20,000 in hilly, desert and difficult terrains) or more population. Each PHC has one medical officer, two health assistants—one male and one female—and health workers and supporting staff. The most peripheral health institutional facility is the sub-centre manned by one male and one female multipurpose health worker. At present, in most places, there is one sub-centre for about 5,000 populations (3,000 in hilly and desert areas and in difficult terrains) (Country Health System Profile: India).

MATERNAL HEALTH IN INDIA: ACHIEVEMENTS AND FAILURES

According to the NFHS-3, 2005–06 (NFHS-3, 2007), maternal and child health has remained an integral part of the Family Welfare Programme of India since the time of the first and second Five-Year Plans (1951–56 and 1956–61) when the Government of India took steps to strengthen maternal and child health services. As part of the Minimum Needs Programme initiated during the fifth Five-Year Plan (1974–79), maternal health, child health and nutrition services were integrated with family planning services. In 1992–93, the Child Survival and Safe Motherhood Programme continued the process of integration by bringing together several key child survival interventions with safe motherhood and family planning activities. In 1996, safe motherhood and child health services were incorporated into the Reproductive and Child Health (RCH) Programme. The National Population Policy adopted by the Government of India in 2000 reiterates the government's commitment to safe motherhood programmes within the wider context of reproductive health. An important objective of NFHS-3, such as NFHS-1 and NFHS-2, was to provide information on the use of safe motherhood services provided by the public and private sectors. The topics covered included pregnancy complications, antenatal and postnatal care, place of and assistance during delivery, delivery characteristics and postpartum complications. Unlike NFHS-2 where information on the utilization of maternal services was collected for the last two live births of ever-married women during the three years preceding the survey, NFHS-3 was expanded to include information on all births to women in the last five years. However, in NFHS-3, most of the detailed information on antenatal, delivery and postnatal care was obtained for only the woman's most recent birth during the five years preceding the survey. A brief review of the chapter on 'maternal health' in the NFHS-3 report is given here as it gives us details of the status of maternal health in India in terms of the various constituents of maternal health.

ANTENATAL CARE

According to NFHS-3, antenatal care (ANC) refers to pregnancy-related health care, which is usually provided by a doctor, an auxiliary nurse midwife (ANM) or another health professional. Ideally, ANC should monitor a pregnancy for signs of complications, detect and treat pre-existing and concurrent problems of pregnancy, and provide advice and counselling on preventive care, diet during pregnancy, delivery care, postnatal care and related issues. The main purposes of ANC are to prevent certain complications, such as anaemia, and identify women with established pregnancy complications for treatment or transfer (Pallikadavath et al., 2004: 1147). In India, the RCH Programme aims at providing at least three antenatal check-ups, which should include a weight and blood pressure check, abdominal examination, immunization against tetanus, iron and folic acid (IFA) prophylaxis, as well as anaemia management. The most commonly reported pregnancy-related health problems are excessive fatigue (48 per cent) and swelling of the legs, body or face (25 per cent). Ten per cent of mothers had convulsions that were not from fever and 9 per cent reported night blindness. Only 4 per cent had any vaginal bleeding.

COMPONENTS OF ANC

The important elements of ANC include the provision of iron supplementation for pregnant mothers, two doses of tetanus toxoid vaccine and a drug to get rid of intestinal worms. Nutritional deficiencies in women are often exacerbated during pregnancy because of the additional nutrient requirements of foetal growth. Iron-deficiency anaemia is the most common micronutrient deficiency in the world. The provision of IFA tablets to pregnant women to prevent nutritional anaemia forms an integral part of the safe motherhood services offered as part of the RCH programme in India. The programme recommendation is that women consume 100 tablets of IFA during pregnancy. The survey revealed that 65 per cent of mothers received IFA supplements for their most recent birth. IFA coverage was well below average for older women, women with fourth or higher order births, women with no education, Muslim women and women in households in the lowest wealth quintile. IFA coverage was also lower in rural areas (61 per cent) than in urban areas (76 per cent).

ANC PROVIDER

More than three-quarters of women in India received ANC for their most recent birth during the five years preceding the survey. Utilization of ANC services for the most recent birth among ever-married women increased substantially over time, from 66 per cent in NFHS-2 to 77 per cent in NFHS-3. The rate of increase was higher in rural areas than in urban areas. In NFHS-3, half of the women received ANC from doctors and 23 per cent received ANC from ANM nurses, midwives or lady health visitors (LHVs). Older women (aged 35–49 years) were much less likely than younger women to have received ANC for their most recent birth, and the likelihood of receiving ANC declined sharply with birth order. Eighty-eight per cent of mothers of first-order births received ANC, compared with only 48 per cent of mothers of births of order six or higher. Ninety-eight per cent of women with 12 or more years of education received ANC compared with 62 per cent of women with no education.

DISPARITIES IN ANC

Almost one out of every five women in India did not receive any ANC for their last birth in the five years preceding the survey. Women not receiving ANC tend disproportionately to be older women, women having children of higher birth orders, scheduled tribe women, women with no education and women in households with a low-wealth index. The utilization of ANC services differed greatly by state: Goa, Kerala and Tamil Nadu ranked among the top five states in the country in terms of their performance on almost all of the indicators. Kerala and Tamil Nadu each ranked highest on four of the nine indicators. Other states that performed relatively well on most of the indicators included Andhra Pradesh, Sikkim, Karnataka, Maharashtra, West Bengal, Punjab, Delhi, Gujarat and Himachal Pradesh. Bihar ranked the lowest on many of the ANC indicators. Arunachal Pradesh, Nagaland, Uttar Pradesh, Jharkhand and Rajasthan also performed poorly on most of the indicators. Compared with Tamil Nadu, for example, where 96 per cent of mothers had three or more ANC visits, only 17 per cent of mothers in Bihar and 27 per cent in Uttar Pradesh had three or more visits. In general, the southern and western states and some of the northern states performed uniformly well. The performance of states in the North-

East region was mixed; notably, however, except for Sikkim and Manipur, the percentage receiving tetanus toxoid injections was below the national average in all of these states.

ANC SERVICES AND INFORMATION

The effectiveness of ANC in ensuring safe motherhood depends, in part, on the medical tests and measurements done and the advice given as part of ANC. Among women receiving ANC for their most recent birth, 72 per cent had an abdominal examination, 64 per cent had their blood pressure checked and 63 per cent had their weight measured. Blood and urine tests were conducted for 60 and 58 per cent of women, respectively. All of these measurements or tests were much more likely to be performed for women in urban areas, younger women (below 35 years of age), women having lower-order births, more educated women, Jain and Sikh women, women in households in the higher wealth quintile, and women who were not from scheduled castes, scheduled tribes or other backward classes. Further, the report suggests that most women did not receive information on specific pregnancy complications, and they were not given advice on where to go if they experienced pregnancy complications.

DETERMINANTS OF ANC

Pallikadavath et al. (2004) reviewed the various determinants of ANC in India. According to them, in developing countries, uptake of ANC is determined by socio-economic factors, demographic factors and availability and access to health facilities. In many parts of the developing world, women's education was found to be an important predictor of ANC utilization. Even in India, a relationship between maternal education and utilization of ANC is evident in many studies (see Bhatia and Cleland, 1995). Studies reveal that education and literacy of women play an important role in achieving improvements in ANC in India. Demographic factors such as order of pregnancy (or number of children), marital status, maternal age and marital duration are reported to have an influence on the utilization of ANC. In India, utilization of ANC was low among women with higher-order pregnancies (Chandrashekar et al., 1998). Other relevant variables according to Pallikadavath et al. (2004) are unmarried status, unions of very short duration, desire for large families, never-use of family planning and unwanted pregnancies. In India, reduced ANC use was noted among women aged under 18 years (Bhatia and Cleland, 1995). Lack of knowledge about antenatal services is an important reason for non-utilization in the northern states of India (Misra et al., 1998). Further, variations in service use are also related to availability and accessibility of care. Pallikadavath et al. (2004) also found religion and caste as two important social factors that influence social practices including belief systems surrounding pregnancy. However, these do not follow a stereotypical pattern (Bhatia and Cleland, 1995).

PLACE OF DELIVERY

The NFHS-3 (2007) provides estimated details of place of delivery for live births in India for five years preceding the survey conducted in 2005–06. Around 38.6 per cent of births in India took place in health facilities. Slightly more than 50 per cent took place in the woman's own home and 9 per cent took place in the parents' home. Births in health facilities were about equally divided between those that took place in a private health facility and those that took place in public institutions (such as government-operated district, *tehsil/taluk*, town or municipal hospitals and PHCs). Two-thirds (67.4 per cent) of deliveries in urban areas and 29 per cent of deliveries in rural areas took place in health facilities. Institutional deliveries, particularly in private sector facilities, increased sharply with the mother's education and with the household wealth index. Hulton et al. (2007) reviewed the quality of maternal health services and considered quality as an important determinant of institutional delivery. For them, a policy emphasis on increasing the rate of childbirth in hospitals inherently assumes that institutions provide an optimal level of care. Referring to several other studies, they suggest that women receive and experience appalling care in some institutions in the developing world (Hulton et al., 2007). They suggest that there is growing evidence that avoidable factors, missed opportunities and substandard care contribute to deaths (Pattinson, 2003; Pitchforth et al., 2006); alongside the continued high levels of mortality and disability, worldwide evidence is emerging to show that the care process itself is dehumanized in many parts of the world; staff are indifferent and uncaring; and there is a lack of privacy, dignity and communication (Miller et al., 2003).

ASSISTANCE DURING DELIVERY

Obstetric care from a trained provider during delivery is recognized as critical for the reduction of maternal and neonatal mortality. Forty-seven per cent of births in the five years preceding the survey were assisted by health personnel, including 35 per cent by a doctor and 10 per cent by an ANM, nurse, midwife or LHV. More than one-third of births (37 per cent) were assisted by a traditional birth attendant (TBA), and 16 per cent were assisted by only friends, relatives or other persons. The percentage of births assisted by a doctor was lower for mothers aged 35–49 years than for younger mothers, and the percentage decreased sharply by birth order. Eighty-one per cent of births to mothers who completed at least 12 years of education were assisted by a doctor, compared with only 16 per cent of births to mothers with no education. Similarly, 12 per cent of births to women in the lowest wealth quintile households were assisted by a doctor, compared with 78 per cent of births to women in households in the highest wealth quintile. Based on mothers' reports, 9 per cent of the children born in India in the five years before the survey were delivered by caesarean section. The proportion of deliveries by caesarean section was three times as high in urban areas (17 per cent) as in rural areas (6 per cent). A total of 28 per cent of deliveries in private health facilities and 15 per cent of deliveries in public sector health facilities were by caesarean section. There is a positive relationship between deliveries conducted by caesarean section and both the educational level of the mother and the household wealth index.

POSTNATAL CARE

The health of a mother and her newborn child depends not only on the health care she receives during her pregnancy and delivery but also on the care she and the infant receive during the first few weeks after delivery. Postnatal check-ups soon after the delivery are particularly important for births that take place in non-institutional settings. Recognizing the importance of postnatal check-ups, the RCH Programme recommends three postnatal visits. The NFHS-3 (2007) report reveals that every woman who had a birth in the five years preceding the survey was asked whether she had massive vaginal bleeding or a very high fever—both symptoms of possible postpartum complications—at any time during the two months after delivery of her most recent child. Women reported massive vaginal bleeding for 12 per cent of births and a very high fever for 14 per cent of births. Both complications were more common among rural than urban mothers. The likelihood of having massive vaginal bleeding did not vary much by place of delivery, but very high fever was much more common for home births than for institutional births. Both complications are somewhat lower than average for births assisted by a doctor.

MATERNAL CARE INDICATORS BY STATE

For India as a whole, mothers of only 15 per cent of births received all of the required components of ANC. This indicator ranges from a high of 64 per cent in Kerala and 56 per cent in Goa to a low of only 2 per cent in Nagaland and 4 per cent in Uttar Pradesh. Other states that performed almost as poor as Uttar Pradesh and Nagaland on this indicator included Bihar, Arunachal Pradesh, Madhya Pradesh, Jharkhand, Meghalaya, Rajasthan and Mizoram, where only 6–9 per cent of the women received the recommended components of ANC. Kerala, followed closely by Goa, also outperformed all other states in terms of delivery care, with nearly all deliveries taking place in medical institutions and a similarly high percentage of deliveries assisted by a health professional. Tamil Nadu, with 88 per cent of births delivered in medical institutions and 91 per cent assisted by a health professional, ranked third among the states on these delivery care indicators. By contrast, only 12–20 per cent of births were delivered in medical institutions in Nagaland, Chhattisgarh, Jharkhand and Bihar. Only 25–29 per cent of deliveries were assisted by health professionals in Nagaland, Uttar Pradesh, Jharkhand and Bihar.

NEW PROGRAMMES AND INITIATIVES

National Rural Health Mission (2005–12)

The Government of India, Ministry of Health and Family Welfare, launched National Rural Health Mission (NRHM) in 2005. It recognizes the importance of health as a contributor of social and economic development and adopts the synergistic approach by relating health to the determinants of good health. It seeks to provide effective health care to rural population with special focus on 18 states, which have weak public health indicators. The core strategies are (i) to train and enhance capacity of Panchayati Raj Institutions (PRIs) to own, control and manage public health services; (ii) promote health care at household through female health activist (Accredited Social Health

Activist or ASHA; (iii) health plan for each village through Village Health Committee of the Panchayat; (iv) strengthening sub-centres through unified fund; and (v) implementation of an inter-sectoral District Health Plan. The supplementary strategies are (i) to regulate private sector including the informal rural practitioners; (ii) to ensure availability of quality services to citizens at reasonable cost; (iii) to promote public–private partnerships; (iv) mainstreaming Ayurveda, Yoga and Naturopathy, Unani, Sidha and Homeopathy (AYUSH); (v) reorienting medical education to support rural health; and (vi) pooling and social health insurance to provide health security.

The NRHM has identified specific goals and objectives to be completed within a time frame. The most important initiative related to maternal health is recruitment of a new category of health worker. According to the Mission Document of NRHM, every village/large habitat will have a female ASHA—chosen by and accountable to the *panchayat*—to act as the interface between the community and the public health system. ASHA would act as a bridge between the ANM and the village and be accountable to the Panchayat. She will be an honorary volunteer, receiving performance-based compensation for promoting universal immunization, referral and escort services for RCH, construction of household toilets and other health care delivery programmes. She will be trained on a pedagogy of public health developed and mentored through a Standing Mentoring Group at national level incorporating best practices and implemented through active involvement of community health resource organizations. She will facilitate preparation and implementation of the Village Health Plan along with *Anganwadi* worker (AWW), ANM, functionaries of other departments and self-help group members, under the leadership of the Village Health Committee of the Panchayat.

ASHA will be promoted all over the country, with special emphasis on the 18 high focus states. The Government of India will bear the cost of training, incentives and medical kits. The remaining components will be funded under Financial Envelope given to the states under the programme. She will be given a drug kit containing generic AYUSH and allopathic formulations for common ailments. The drug kit would be replenished from time to time. Induction training of ASHA will be for 23 days in all, spread over 12 months, and on-the-job training would continue throughout the year. It also talks about prototype training material and cascade model of training proposed through training of trainers including contract plus distance learning model. The training would require partnership with NGOs/ ICDS Training Centres and State Health Institutes. According to a Ministry of Health and Family Welfare Report, 7.49 lakh ASHAs were selected and 7.05 lakh ASHAs were trained in the first module by 2010 (MoHFW, 2010).

Janani Suraksha Yojana

Janani Suraksha Yojana (JSY) is a safe motherhood intervention under the NRHM being implemented with the objective of reducing maternal and neonatal mortality by promoting institutional delivery among the poor pregnant women. The Yojana, launched on 12 April 2005, is being implemented in all states and Union Territories with special focus on low-performing states (LPS). It is a 100 per cent centrally sponsored scheme, and it integrates cash assistance with delivery and post-delivery care. The indicator of success of the scheme is the increase in institutional delivery among the poor families. The Yojana has identified ASHA as an effective link between the government and the poor pregnant women in 10 LPS, namely the 8 Empowered Action Group (EAG) states and Assam and Jammu and Kashmir and the remaining North-Eastern states. In other eligible states and Union Territories, wherever AWW and TBA or ASHA-like activist has been engaged in this purpose, she can be associated with this Yojana for providing the services. The scheme focuses on poor pregnant women with special dispensation for states having low institutional delivery rates, namely Uttar Pradesh, Uttaranchal, Bihar, Jharkhand, Madhya Pradesh, Chhattisgarh, Assam, Rajasthan, Odisha and Jammu and Kashmir. Although these states have been named as LPS, the remaining states have been named as high-performing states. Each beneficiary registered under this Yojana should have a JSY. For ASHA/AWW/any other identified link worker under the overall supervision of the ANM and the MO, PHC should mandatorily prepare a micro-birth plan. This will effectively help in monitoring antenatal check-up, and post delivery care. Under this programme, the delivering mother and the recommending ASHA from rural areas will get cash assistance of ₹ 1,400 and ₹ 600 respectively, after the first and second institutional delivery. The amount for the urban areas is ₹ 1,000 and ₹200 respectively.

Rashtriya Swasthya Bima Yojana

Rashtriya Swasthya Bima Yojana (RSBY) was launched by the Ministry of Labour and Employment, Government of India, on 1 April 2008 to provide health insurance coverage for Below Poverty Line (BPL) families. The objective of RSBY is to provide protection to BPL households from financial liabilities arising out of health shocks that involve hospitalization. Beneficiaries under RSBY are entitled to hospitalization coverage up to ₹ 30,000 for most of the diseases that require hospitalization. Government has even fixed the package rates for the hospitals for a large number of interventions. Pre-existing conditions are covered from day 1 and there is no age limit. Coverage extends to five members of the family, which includes the head of household, spouse and up to three dependents. Beneficiaries need to pay only ₹ 30 as registration fee while Central and State Government pays the premium to the insurer selected by the State Government on the basis of a competitive bidding.

CONSTRAINTS AND LIMITATIONS

Sunil et al. (2006: 1944–45) reviewed the research related to utilization of maternal care services in rural India and found that there are many limitations of such services: Although prior studies on utilization of maternal care in India have focused on individual characteristics (Bhatia and Cleland, 1995; Raghupathy, 1996; Navaneetham and Dharmalingam, 2002), the effects of the programme components seldom received any attention. Many studies have approached the use of health care services as a behavioural phenomenon (Becker et al., 1993; Chakraborty et al., 2003), whereas the quality and cost of and access to services are not included. Analysis using the NFHS-1 indicated that community access to health facilities is not an important factor in explaining the utilization of various ANC services (Das et al., 2001). Studies from western societies, however, have often argued that the use of health care services is determined not merely by design and delivery strategies but also by the characteristics of potential users (Andersen and Newman, 1973; Phillips et al., 1998). Thus, the mere existence of health care facilities may not ensure utilization; there is a need to identify the various constraints and limitations in the prevailing health structures and address each of them separately. Some of such constraints are given here. They are applicable for maternal health care as well as general health care.

Limited Budgetary Allocation

Limited budgetary allocation from the central and state governments is a big hurdle. In developed countries, government health spending is around 5 per cent of GDP or more (Norway—6.9 per cent of GDP, USA—6.2 per cent of GDP, etc.). Even in Asian developed countries excluding India, the average health spending is around 3 per cent of GDP. The government health expenditure in India amounts to less than 1 per cent of GDP (these account for less than 20 per cent of the overall health spending). Further, this ratio is not only low internationally but is even lower compared to our own past experience. This low spending on health and the dominance of private sources of financing make India unique. This reflects the very low priority that governments in India have accorded to the health sector (High Level Expert Group, 2011) (for details on health expenditure, see also Khanday and Akram, 2013).

Limited Reach and Scope of Primary Health Care

The other important constraint is limited reach and scope of primary health care in India. Primary health care is the backbone of any health system all over the world. The Alma Ata Declaration (1978) states that primary health care includes at least (i) education concerning prevailing health problems and the methods of preventing and controlling them; (ii) promotion of food supply and proper nutrition; (iii) an adequate supply of safe water and basic sanitation; (iv) maternal and child health care, including family planning; (v) immunization against the major infectious disease; (vi) prevention and control of local endemic disease; (vii) appropriate treatment of common disease and injuries; and (viii) provision of essential drugs. However, most of the elements suggested for primary health care find no mention in the structuring of 'PHCs' in India. If we go back to the Bhore Committee Report submitted in 1946, we find that many of the radical suggestions made by it have never been implemented. The notion of primary health care is an obvious omission. The PHCs in India are understaffed and chronically suffer from the problem of absenteeism and lack of physical resources.

Narrowing of Public Health

The notion of primary health care rests upon the system of 'public health'. The Expert Committee of WHO has defined public health as the

> science and art of preventing diseases, prolonging life and promoting mental and physical health and efficiency through organized community efforts for the sanitation of the environment, the control of communicable infection, the education of the individual's personal hygiene, the organization of medical and nursing services for early diagnosis and preventive treatment of disease, the development of the social machinery to ensure to every individual a standard of living, adequate for the maintenance of health and so organizing these benefits as to enable every citizen to realize his birth right of health and longevity (WHO, 1952).

Public health in India is in a dilapidated condition. The prevalence of communicable diseases at such a vast magnitude is a testimony to it. A large number of maternal mortalities are caused by such communicable diseases. There is no formal identifiable structure for promoting public health in India, and whatever structures existed are getting diluted. The recent coming into existence of the Public Health Foundation of India is more cosmetic than structural (because of the lack of supporting infrastructure and undefined target/resource base). No specific budget is marked for various requirements under public health. Water, sanitation, food, nutrition, adulteration, etc., are not seen from a comprehensive public health perspective. Das Gupta (2005) reviewed the state of public health in India and found several conditions and factors responsible for the poor state of public health in India. Some of these conditions reflect the limitations of public health in contemporary India and most of its states.

The public health successes achieved in the developed world by the late nineteenth and early twentieth centuries meant that by the 1940s, their main causes of death shifted from communicable to non-communicable diseases such as cardiovascular diseases and cancer. Simultaneously, the government's focus shifted from improving public health systems to improving curative technologies and methods of health care financing. Invention of antibiotics is a major breakthrough in curing diseases. Techniques for mass production of antibiotics were refined during the 1940s. This made it possible for local elites (rich) to protect themselves from dying of communicable diseases, without having to maintain rigorous environmental hygiene to prevent exposure to disease for the rich and poor alike. Consequently, the focus of medical research shifted away from finding new technologies for communicable disease control—except when threatened by newly emergent diseases against which they have no protection, such as the avian flu.

An important development of the 1950s is the merger of the public health services with the medical services. Specialization in curative skills became far better rewarded than public health and attracted the best talent. Gradually, senior positions in public health were filled by people with no training or experience in public health. An inconsistency between constitutional provisions starved public health systems of funds in many of the states. Public health services were designated as the responsibility of the state governments, except for issues such as port quarantine and provisions relating to the spread of diseases between states (for a detailed discussion, see Akram, 2013).

Medicalization of All Financial Resources

Medicalization caused substantial proportions of the health budgets to go on expanding subsidized medical training, public sector employment for medical graduates and high-end tertiary medical services—all of which largely benefits the middle classes and detracts from the provision of public and primary health services. One of the consequences of over-medicalization, in India, is narrowing the field of 'primary health care'. Further, health is often used (selectively and consciously) synonymously with medical. In all such situations, all other social and environmental dimensions of health are relegated to the background. Consequently, the very important health components such as the basic health goods (BHGs) become victim of medical (say financial) negligence and 'overlooking' (for a detailed discussion, see Akram, 2012b).

WAY FORWARD

The infrastructure for the delivery of health services grew substantially in post-independent India, and the health of the population gradually improved during the past six decades. India has one of the world's largest networks of health centres and hospitals under a public health system. The private health care is also flourishing. Medical tourism is attracting potential users from other developed nations. The life expectancy in India has increased substantially since independence. But, despite these achievements, India ranked a low of 119th among 169 countries in the 2010 Human Development Index. The out-of-pocket expenditure on health care is pushing the huge population back to the BPL status. The widespread scams and financial irregularities taking place in government funds provided for health care reflect poor administration of the scarce resources. Hence, it is the right time to make evidence-based and conscientious assessment of the health achievements of the past and redesign the future. It is time to realize that the anomalies in the outcome of health and health care are not just the consequence of illiteracy or poverty alone. To a great extent, these are also consequences of cumulative wrongs at the level of policy prioritization and planning.

There is a need to revisit the Alma Ata Declaration of 1978, which gave a comprehensive design for primary health care for achieving the targets of health for all. The PHCs in India are the backbone of the health structure, but such PHCs are unable to translate the goals of primary health care as envisaged by the Alma Ata Declaration. Out of the eight primary elements necessary for primary health care as suggested by the Alma Ata Declaration (1978), the author considers unadulterated nutritious food, safe drinking water and sanitation as the BHGs. BHGs are basic in the sense that they are indispensable for human life, and life is impossible without them. The goal of achieving 'health for all' is just an illusion without the comprehensive and sustainable availability of the BHGs to all individuals in any society, and more particularly in developing societies such as India. Most of the communicable diseases are caused due to the lack of BHGs. Hence, BHGs should be seen as an integral and undisputable component of the health needs of the population in general and women and children in particular. Most of the maternal health complications are also related to unavailability of such BHGs.

The government must increase the allocations for the health budget and the lion's share of this should be given for improving the public health system. The availability of health care centres must be made commensurate with the population density and pressure. The decimal presence of the public health centres forces people to go for private medical care that enhances the cost of medical care many times more. Instead of providing financial incentives for institutional delivery (as under JSY), the government must improve the quality of care, which will automatically attract the needful. The government needs to monitor and regulate the private and especially the corporate sector for checking the ever-increasing prices of the medicines, drugs and surgical corrections. The health coverage through insurance needs proper standardization. Good governance and better administration are very instrumental in achieving health goals within a time frame. Bureaucratic accountability and sensitization is a must for combating the ongoing marginalization and exclusions of the deprived sections. The increasing inequality and disparity in health outcomes needs to be controlled. It is time to make necessary improvements in the health policies and to show a human as well as a humanitarian face of politico-administrative processes in India.

REFERENCES

Advani, M. and M. Akram, 2007, 'Health Concerns in India'. In *Health Dynamics and Marginalized Communities*, edited by M. Akram, Jaipur: Rawat Publications, pp. 3–26.

Akram, M., 2007, 'Introduction'. In *Health Dynamics and Marginalized Communities*, edited by M. Akram, Jaipur: Rawat Publications, pp. ix–xx.

Akram, M., 2012a, 'Challenges before Health Planning in India: Preparing Draft of the 12th Five Year Plan', *Journal of US-China Public Administration*, 9(2): 229–34.

Akram, M., 2012b, 'Looking Beyond the Universal Health Coverage: Health Inequality, Medicalism and Dehealthism in India', *Public Health Research*, 2(6): 221–28, doi: 10.5923/j.phr.20120206.08, [online] available at http://www.sapub.org/global/showpaperpdf.aspx?doi=10.5923/j.phr.20120206.08 (accessed on 5 January 2013).

Akram, M., 2013, *Health Inequality, Basic Health Goods and Dehealthism* (Occasional Paper Series, DRS-I in Sociology, AMU, Aligarh). New Delhi: Icon Publications Pvt. Ltd.

Andersen, R. and J.F. Newman, 1973, 'Societal and Individual Determinants of Medical Care Utilization in the United States', *Milbank Memorial Fund Quarterly*, 51(1): 95–124.

Becker, S., H.P. David, H.G. Ronald, G. Connie and E.B. Robert, 1993, 'The Determinants of Use of Maternal and Child Health Services in Metro Cebu, the Philippines'. *Health Transition Review*, 3(1): 77–89.

Bhatia, J.C. and J. Cleland, 1995, 'Determinants of Maternal Care in a Region of South India', *Health Transition Review*, 5(2): 127–42.

Chakraborty, N., M.A. Islam, R.I. Chowdhury, W. Bari and H.H. Akhter, 2003, 'Determinants of the Use of Maternal Health Services in Rural Bangladesh', *Health Promotion International*, 18(4): 327–37.

Chandrashekar, S., R.S. Phaneendran and N.S. Nair, 1998, 'Socio-demographic Determinants of Antenatal Care', *Tropical Doctor*, 28: 206–09.

Country Health System Profile: India, Year not mentioned, WHO/SEARO, [online] available at http://www.searo.who.int/en/Section313/Section1519_10853.htm (accessed on 9 September 2011).

Das, N.P., V.K. Mishra and P.K. Saha, 2001, 'Does Community Access Affect the Use of Health and Family Welfare Services in Rural India?' *National Family Health Survey Subject Reports*, Number 18.

Das Gupta, M., 2005, *Public Health in India: An Overview*, Development Research Group, World Bank Policy Research Working Paper 3787, The World Bank, December 2005.

High Level Expert Group Report on Universal Health Coverage, 2011, [online] available at http://planningcommission.nic.in/reports/genrep/rep_uhc0812.pdf (accessed on 5 July 2012).

Hulton, L.H., Z. Matthews and R.W. Stones, 2007, 'Applying a Framework for Assessing the Quality of Maternal Health Services in Urban India', *Social Science and Medicine*, 64: 2083–95.

Jeffery, P. and R. Jeffery, 2010, 'Only when the Boat has Started Sinking: A Maternal Death in Rural North India', *Social Science & Medicine*, 71: 1711–18.

Khanday, Z.A. and M. Akram, 2013, 'A Study of Health Structure and Health Expenditure Patterns in Anantnag District of Jammu and Kashmir', *International Journal of Social and Behavioural Sciences*, 1(2): 65–76, [online] available at http://www.academeresearchjournals.org/download.php?id=859435318007570879.pdf&type=application/pdf&op=1 (accessed on 19 February 2013).

MDG-ICR, 2011, Millennium Development Goals-India Country Report, Central Statistical Organization, Ministry of Statistics and Programme Implementation, Government of India, [online] available at http://www.undp.org/content/dam/india/docs/mdg_india_2011.pdf (accessed on 5 July 2012).

Miller, S., M. Cordero, A.L. Coleman, J. Figueroa, S. Brito Anderson, R. Dabagh, V. Calderon, F. Cáceres, A.J. Fernandez and M. Nunez, 2003, 'Quality of Care in Institutionalized Deliveries: The Paradox of the Dominican Republic', *International Journal of Gynecology and Obstetrics*, 82(1): 89–103.

Ministry of Health and Family Welfare, 2010, *The Journey so far 2005–10, NRHM: Meeting People's Health Needs in Partnership with States*. New Delhi: Government of India.

Misra, U.S., T.K. Roy and S. Rajan Irudaya, 1998, 'Antenatal Care and Contraceptive Behaviour in India: Some Evidence from the National Family Health Survey', *The Journal of Family Welfare*, 44: 1–14.

Navaneetham, K. and A. Dharmalingam, 2002, 'Utilization of Maternal Health Care Services in Southern India', *Social Science & Medicine*, 55: 1849–69.

NFHS-3, 2007, *National Family Health Survey (NFHS-3), 2005–06: India: Volume I*. Mumbai: International Institute for Population Sciences (IIPS) and Macro International.

Pallikadavath, S., M. Foss and R.W. Stones, 2004, 'Antenatal Care: Provision and Inequality in Rural North India', *Social Science & Medicine*, 59: 1147–58.

Pattinson, R.C., 2003, 'Challenges in Saving Babies—Avoidable Factors, Missed Opportunities and Substandard Care in Perinatal Deaths in South Africa', *South African Medical Journal*, 3(6): 450–55.

Phillips, K.A., K.R. Morrison, R. Andersen and L.A. Aday, 1998, 'Understanding the Context of Health Care Utilization: Assessing Environmental and Provider-Related Variables in the Behavioral Model of Utilization', *Health Services Research*, 33(3): 571–96.

Pitchforth, E., E. van Teijlingen, W. Graham, M. Dixon-Woods and M. Chowdhury, 2006, 'Getting Women to Hospital is not Enough', *Quality and Safety in Health Care*, 15: 214–19.

Raghupathy, S., 1996, 'Education and the use of Maternal Health Care in Thailand', *Social Science and Medicine*, 43(4): 459–71.

Sample Registration System (SRS), 2011, Maternal and Child Mortality and Total Fertility Rates, Office of Registrar General, India, [online] available at http://censusindia.gov.in/vital_statistics/SRS_Bulletins/MMR_release_070711.pdf (accessed on 3 July 2012).

Sunil, T.S., S. Rajaram and L.K. Zottarelli, 2006, 'Do Individual and Program Factors Matter in the Utilization of Maternal Care Services in Rural India? A Theoretical Approach', *Social Science and Medicine*, 62: 1943–57.

The Declaration of Alma-Ata, 1978, [online] available at http://www.who.int/social_determinants/tools/multimedia/alma_ata/en/index.html (accessed on 14 July 2012).

United Nations, 1948, *Documents*, [online] available at http://www.un.org/en/documents/udhr/ (accessed on 5 July 2012).

WHO, 1952, *Report of Expert Committee on Public Health Administration*. Geneva: WHO/SEARO.

WHO, 1996, *Care in Normal Birth: A Practical Guide*. Geneva: WHO/FRH/MSM 96–24.

WHO, 2005, *Improving Maternal, Newborn and Child Health in the South-East Asia Region*, [online] available at www.searo.who.int/en/Section260/Section1808/Section1933.htm (accessed on 5 July 2012).

WHO, 2006, *Defining Sexual Health: Report of a Technical Consultation on Sexual Health*, Geneva, [online] available at http://www.who.int/reproductivehealth/publications/sexual_health/defining_sexual_health.pdf (accessed on 5 July 2012).

WHO, 2009, *Women and Health: Today's Evidence Tomorrow's Agenda*, [online] available at http://whqlibdoc.who.int/publications/2009/9789241563857_eng.pdf (accessed on 5 July 2012).

WHO, 2011, *International Statistical Classification of Diseases and Related Health Problems*, 10th revision (ICD-10), volume 2, Instruction manual, 2010 edition, WHO, p. 156, [online] available at http://www.who.int/classifications/icd/en/index.html (accessed on 5 July 2012).

WHO, 2012, *Trends in Maternal Mortality: 1990 to 2010*. Geneva, WHO, UNICEF, UNFPA and The World Bank Estimates.

CHAPTER 2

Understanding Women's Health and Rights Issues

Madhu Nagla

INTRODUCTION

The concept of right to health as a human right has recently emerged as a result of ever-growing consciousness about the dignity of human life across the world. Health care is considered as a socio-medical concept, which implies that whatever is medically possible to promote the physical, mental and well-being of the patient must be done. Medical profession, which is a noble profession, has now become a business. Medical professionals often forget their responsibilities towards their patients and conduct their professional work without observing the code of ethics, and thereby violate the rights of the patients. Growing incidences of malpractice and medical negligence on the part of medical professionals result in poor health or sometimes in medical complications of the patients. Because women constitute nearly half of the population of any country and possess an additional responsibility of reproduction and motherhood, they are obviously more likely to be a victim of improper health care.

Before any treatment or investigation, patients have the right to a clear, concise explanation in lay terms of the proposed procedure and of any available alternative procedure. Wherever applicable the explanation shall incorporate information on risks, side effects or aftereffects, problems relating to recuperation, likelihood of success, risk of death and whether the proposed procedure is to be administered by or in the presence of students.

If a patient is in a hospital or any other health care facility, the patient shall, unless incapacitated, be consulted about any decision with respect to discharge or transfer to another facility. Where it is appropriate to a patient's condition or treatment, the patient should be given advice about self-care, drug administration and special precautions that may be necessary or desirable, and the existence of special association, facilities, aids or appliances that may be of assistance. A patient's consent should be obtained before any procedure is carried out. A patient may refuse any treatment or investigation at any given period. No patient should be treated or examined without his or her consent. If a patient is incapacitated and delay would be dangerous, a doctor is entitled to carry out any necessary treatment or operation. A patient's written consent should be obtained for his or her inclusion in any research. The patient should be adequately informed of the aims, methods, anticipated benefits and potential hazards of the study and the discomfort it may entail. The patient should be informed that he or she is free to withdraw his or her consent to participation at any time. To ensure that the informed consent is not obtained under duress or from a patient in a dependent relationship to the health professional, the informed consent should be obtained by a health professional who is not engaged in the investigation and who is completely independent of the official relationship between the patient and the health professional.

According to the human rights, which guarantees equality between sexes, many of the health disadvantages of women can be put under scrutiny. Gender disparities that affect many women have led to a host of health problems including unintended pregnancy, family planning methods, breastfeeding and sex-selective technology. Gender consideration often leads to denial of various human rights including the access to adequate information regarding sterilization in family planning, sex-selective amniocentesis test, breastfeeding and access to safe abortion. The present paper focuses on the understanding of women's rights to health issues in the context of the above-mentioned issues.

Human life is precious, and every person has a fundamental right to live with dignity. It is the duty of a welfare state to protect and develop the life of every citizen and to promote his or her rights to health and medical care. Right to medical care is important because it relates to the very existence of human life. Medical care is as essential as the other basic needs of a person such as food, water, shelter and clothing. Every nation has evolved its own system of laws to ensure the health rights of its citizens. These laws aim at establishing a humane system of health care based on the principles of equity, justice and efficiency. By emphasizing the rights of the citizens for proper health care, the welfare government tries to enhance the welfare of its people so that they can live healthy and predictive lives.

Right to health and health care is also a fundamental right under Article 21 of the Constitution of India. This has also been emphasized by the Supreme Court of India in several obligations on the state to protect citizen's life from medical and other forms of negligence. Although the Consumer Protection Act is applicable across India, it does not fall under the category of state-level health legislation.

CONTEXT

Reproductive health is a matter of concern for women. There are several facets to it. Decision to conceive the child, the use of different family planning methods, breastfeeding and nuances of sex-selective technology are some of the concerns that are exclusively related to women vis-à-vis her health. This chapter focuses on the emerging health right issues concerned with women. In the light of the above concerns, we try to address the following issues:

1. What is the nature of health complications and procedures associated with family planning, sex-determination test, breastfeeding and abortion?
2. How are health rights conflicting with women's issues of health care?

METHODOLOGY

An interview forms an extremely interesting and rich source of information, and it makes the research process thoroughly realistic. We have also tried to present the feel of the fieldwork experience by allowing the voices of some of those whom we interviewed in the context of their autonomy and rights in the different health facilities.

The following sections present the account of visits to a family planning clinic in the Outpatient Department (OPD) of a medical college hospital and private health facilities during our study. The present paper is based on a larger study (Nagla, 2007) on the various facets of the gender inequality of health in which some ethnographic and health narratives are also one of the components. The data of the study were collected during April–June 2006. I was there during clinic hours, and the women attending the clinic were being seen throughout the interview. For me, it turned out to be as much as an occasion to observe as to conduct an interview. The analysis of the present study is based on some case studies gathered during the fieldwork done in relation to women with their health concerns in the city of Rohtak, Haryana. The empirical evidences are presented in the form of narratives gathered from the women during our fieldwork. The paper seeks to discuss some of these questions in the context of evidence on the understanding of women and their rights in different areas of their health concern.

WOMEN STERILIZATION (FAMILY PLANNING METHOD)

Human rights activists demand that choosing a contraceptive and the type of contraceptive or discontinuing contraceptive use should be the individual woman's decision and not that of the medical personnel who provide medical service. Providers of contraceptive technologies believe in the principle of free and informed choice; but, in practice, they often do not adhere to it, stating that they are more aware of what is good for the individual in question. Choices should be based on sufficient and unbiased information. The doctor should provide information about all methods (including barrier methods and natural methods, access to safe abortion and sterilization), how to use them, their advantages and disadvantages in terms of both efficacy and adverse effects (health risks) and allow an individual to choose the method once medical contra-indications have been established. Unbalanced and incomplete information may be falsely reassuring and thereby lead to inappropriate use and possible hazard to women (Gupta, 2000).

The most common method of contraception used in India, besides abortion, is sterilization, of which the majority is that of female sterilization. During the 1960s and early 1970s, vasectomy was promoted in India's family planning programme. Since then, at policy level, vasectomy has been almost totally replaced by tubectomy. India has started payment of incentives particularly after vasectomy since the mid-1960s. This was considered a compensation for loss of wages for staying away from work for about five days. Paid leave after voluntary sterilization is given in India to government employees. There are some state and central government employees who are given advance increments, loans with low interest rates, etc., after voluntary sterilization, of course with lower age and parity restrictions. Cash incentives to the motivators and/or to the providers of services, for example, surgeons, nurses and other paramedical staff after voluntary sterilization are also given. Laparoscopic sterilizations are often done in sub-optimal conditions, in either institutional or mobile settings. In rural areas, camps are organized in temporary locations such as school buildings or some other public facility on special occasions. In these camps, a single surgeon performs 300–500 laparoscopies in 10 hours per day, which works out to one operation every two minutes. With the minimal care that is necessary for such an operation, only a maximum of 50 laparoscopies a day would be possible (Gupta, 2000). In Kumbakonam, 1,225 women were operated in one day (Balasurbrahmanyan, 1986). In such a setting, it must be expected that the attitude of the health personnel would be callous. Obviously, follow-up care is not part of such mass programmes, which provide the facility of sterilization and move on. Often these areas do not have hospitals or clinics where women who have problems can go for help.

Ramanathan et al. (1995) note that 48 sterilizations were performed by one surgical team in just over two hours, which is a clear violation of the regulations. Counselling of women before the operation was inadequate, the surgeon never changed his gloves, the linen on the operating tables was never changed and the facilities in the building were grossly insufficient to support post-operation requirements.

Malini Karkal mentions 'a study of 9,066 laparoscopies conducted in camps over 10 years reported surgical difficulties for 7.9% of the clients, complications for 5.3%, and failure rates of 0.6 per 100 women years. The Indian Association of Gynecological Endoscopists has registered its concern for the use of this method' (Karkal, 1985: 39). Padma Prakash (1984) reports a death rate of 10–12 per 100,000 laparoscopic sterilizations, compared to an acceptable figure of 0.25–0.5. The Indian Association of Gynaecological Endoscopists issued a strong statement criticizing the way mass sterilization camps are conducted. Some even condemned the way of working of such 'professional laparoscopists' and their 'craze for speed' and the setting of daily targets, which have resulted in both 'method failure' and medical complications for women (Prakash, 1984). The providers of the services, that is doctors themselves, were not aware of the standards, and the quality of the services provided by them was found to be poor in all locations (Rajya Sabha, 2003). Mavalankar and Sharma (1999) in their study of sterilization in camps of Gujarat found that many potential clients are reluctant to undergo sterilization despite not wanting more children because of poor quality of care.

Unnithan-Kumar (2003) found that there is a widespread belief among Darana women and men as well as in the surrounding villages that even when you go to public hospital to have a child, the doctors perform tubectomies (effectively terminating women's ability to conceive). Middle-class, high-caste doctors force poor, low-caste women to undergo sterilization with no thought for women's own choices, desires or even their past reproductive histories. This is also evident in Ram's study (1998) of the relationship between maternity and modernity in Tamil Nadu.

Recently (*The Times of India*, 2012), a surgeon in Bihar's Araria district on January 7 conducted 53 sterilization operations on women in two hours with the help of unqualified staff in Kaparfora Government Middle School that did not have basic amenities such as running water or sterilizing equipment. It is a clear violation of nearly all the guidelines, because neither the NGO nor the surgeon conducted pre-operative tests to determine suitability of the enlisted women for sterilization. As a result of these operations, three women were left profusely bleeding. Another woman was operated despite being three months pregnant. She miscarried days after the procedure. After the surgeries, all the 53 women were crying out in pain. Although they were in desperate need of medical care, no one came to assist them.

The situation in government hospitals and family welfare clinics is no better. Our study also observed a specific situation in the field setting. We interviewed the women to know about the details of entering into hospital up to the follow-up procedure, and we found that more than 70 per cent women were illiterate. These illiterate women were not able to read and write, therefore, their signing of consent form for their sterilization is under question. They were neither informed nor counselled for their sterilization in relation to the wider choices of different methods. There is a clear violation of the directions of the guidelines as well as violation of Section 90 of the Indian Penal Code relating to informed consent, in the way sterilization camps were conducted. The women are only informed that tubectomy is the best method, and therefore, they perform tubectomy on the women for their goodness. Before sterilization, it is mandatory that the doctor analyses the history of the patient to determine whether the patient is compatible for sterilization or not. However, the history that is taken is restricted only to the menstrual and obstetric history, and nothing more than that. The physical examination of pelvic is also done in a causal manner without bothering to change gloves for each patient. Urine examination and haemoglobin examination are done in a routine manner. There is no cleanliness of toilets, and therefore, there are chances of infection that can get transmitted from one person to another. The operating surgeons do not conduct any final assessment of the women before performing sterilization. There are no cases of refusal of sterilization on the basis of relative contradiction, clinical assessment or laboratory examination in the health care facility.

In the context of sterilization, informed consent means that the patient is aware of the other choices of methods of contraception besides the possible health problems that might occur and gives her consent voluntarily without any inducement, force, deceit, bias or any other form of coercion. The informed consent of the individual acceptor is a must in case of voluntary sterilization. The consent may be considered informed if the person consenting had the full information on the following:

1. The nature of operation
2. Its consequences, risks and the possibility that it may not succeed
3. Availability of an alternative to voluntary sterilization

The above information can also be given by the paramedical staff apart from the doctors.

In view of the prevalent gender norms that rationalize the bargaining power of women, lack of informed choice and high infant as well as child mortality, female sterilization as a family planning measure in India raises questions about the rights of women.

Clients must be told that women have the option of deciding against the procedure at any time without sacrificing their right to other reproductive health services. The client must be told that a reversal of this surgery is possible, but the reversal involves a major surgery and its success cannot be guaranteed. Consent for sterilization operation should not be obtained under coercion or when the client is under physical or mental stress. Consent should not be obtained when a woman is sedated or when she experiences stress associated with some pregnancy-related events/problems. Clients must sign a printed application and consent form for sterilization. There are certain conditions that require doctors to be cautious, delay the surgery, refer the client to a specialty-equipped centre or counsel to opt for alternative contraception. There may be situations when it is better to counsel the client's husband to go in for vasectomy. There are no absolute contra-indications for tubectomy. Temporary contra-indications include anaemia, severe hypertension, diabetes, local skin diseases, etc. The best timing for performing tubectomy is even after delivery, and it is called postpartum sterilization. Tubectomy can also be performed after periods when pregnancy is ruled out. This procedure is called interval tubectomy or tubectomy can be done after the woman undergoes medical termination of pregnancy (MTP) or spontaneous abortion. Female sterilization by minilap tubectomy can be performed by a trained MBBS doctor, whereas laparoscopic sterilization can be performed either by a gynaecologist with DGO/MD/MS or by a surgeon trained in laparoscopy with an MS degree. Prior to performing sterilization, a careful clinical assessment of the clients should be made to ensure their fitness for surgery. Tubectomy is done by either laparotomy, which entails opening of the abdomen by a small incision, or laparoscopy. Tubectomy by laparotomy is best done in the postpartum period when the operation is quite simple to perform as the uterus at this stage is quite large. This is a very simple and safe procedure. The operation is done at least 24 hours after delivery so that the woman has adequate rest and has sufficient time to make up her mind as this is a permanent procedure. Her haemoglobin and urine are checked preoperatively. Consent of the woman is enough for this operation. Husband's consent is not a must for this operation. The operating doctor confirms her physical fitness for this operation before proceeding for the surgery. Tubectomy can be performed under local, spinal or general anaesthesia. Preparation for surgery includes preoperative assessment and instructions, a review of the surgical procedure and 24 post-operative care. Preoperative assessment is essential to assess the client's physical fitness for surgery and also ensure that the consent for surgery is voluntary and well informed. This assessment can also provide an opportunity for overall health screening and treatment of reproductive tract infection (RTI)/sexually transmitted diseases (STDs), if required demographic information on age, marital status, occupation, religion, education, number of living children, sex and age of the youngest child is required to be elicited.

Women are often provided inadequate time and information for-consent to sterilization procedures, or are never told or discover later that they have been sterilized.

One of the women reported that:

> She had four children when she visited the family planning centre for some method of contraception. She did not want to have any children. She asked the doctor to help her out for the conception. The doctor advised her to go for sterilization without suggesting any other method. She agreed for sterilization. After sterilization now she is having frequent problems of backache, menstrual cycle problem and weakness.

Another woman shared:

> I delivered a third child and doctor asked me to go immediately for sterilization. I along with my husband and my family members gave the consent for the same. After two days of sterilization, I had many complications. Doctors were unable to treat me properly. I still feel that I could have managed birth control without sterilization method.

Regarding the choice of method of family planning one woman said:

> I completed my family planning and I am using Copper-T all through years. However after three years I went to family planning for removing the Copper-T as I was having some problems. I asked the doctors to suggest me some other methods as I turned 42 years. The doctor forcefully advised me for sterilization. I had sterilization, again I am having health problems.

Thus, in relation to women and the family planning programme there is a blatant flouting; the procedures for sterilizations, avoidance of informed consent and follow-up of sterilization cases are likely to have a serious long-term consequences on women's health. Abortion is linked with sterilization in government facility, thus ignoring the rights of women.

WOMEN AND SEX-SELECTION AMNIOCENTESIS TEST

Amniocentesis was first introduced in India in 1974 at the All-India Institute of Medical Sciences (AIIMS), New Delhi, to detect foetal abnormalities. By 1975, it was known that the test was being used for conducting sex-selective abortion. However, sex determination was banned, first in 1988 in Maharashtra and then in other parts of the country. This ban did not stop the lucrative business of sex-determination tests; rather, it spread into all parts of the country. It was found that there was violation of medical ethics by medical personnel in using technologies that were principally meant for detecting genetic abnormalities for determining the sex of the foetus, and further misusing the liberal abortion laws of the country by performing sex-selective abortions (Gupta, 2000).

The amniocentesis procedure is usually performed between 14 and 20 weeks and sometimes as early as 11 weeks of pregnancy. In some cases, amniocentesis may be performed in the third trimester. Amniocentesis is carried out to determine uterine infections in the case of ruptured membranes. It also helps determine feral anaemia in babies with Rhesus (Rh) disease. In such cases, it also helps the doctor to decide whether the foetus requires blood transfusions to save its life. During the third trimester, amniocentesis also helps assessing lung maturity. Amniocentesis is considered to be a safe procedure, but as it is an invasive diagnostic test, it has its own share of risks. There are some amniocentesis risks that should be noted before carrying out the procedure. These risks include the following:

1. **Miscarriage**: The rate of amniocentesis risks of miscarriage is about 1 in 300 to 1 in 500. The amniocentesis risks of miscarriage are high if carried out before 14 weeks of pregnancy. Miscarriages happen due to infection in the uterus, the water breaks or labour is induced prematurely. Amniocentesis risks for twins or multiple pregnancies are the same as the slight risk of miscarriage in normal pregnancies.
2. **Cramps and Vaginal Bleeding**: Another risk of amniocentesis in some women is cramping and vaginal bleeding.
3. **Foetal Injury**: In extremely rare cases, the needle comes in contact with the baby. This may happen in case the baby moves an arm or leg and comes in contact with the needle. It is very rare to observe serious needle injuries in foetus while performing amniocentesis.
4. **Rh Sensitization**: Again in rare cases, the foetal blood cells enter the mother's bloodstream triggering an immune response. This happens when the mother is Rh negative and the foetus has Rh positive blood group. In such cases, the doctor may give the mother

Rh immunoglobulin drugs to prevent production of antibodies against the foetal blood cells.

5. **Uterine Infections**: Sometimes, amniocentesis may trigger a uterine infection that may lead to miscarriage. If the mother has hepatitis B or C, it may increase the risk of transmission to baby in the first or second trimesters. Amniocentesis also increases the risk of HIV from the mother being transmitted to the baby. Thus, one should avoid it in the third trimester.

Some other side effects of amniocentesis include leakage of fluid and minor irritation at the puncture site.

The following reportings by women will make us understand that they are not informed about the health problems resulting out of the amniocentesis test:

> One of the women reported that she had gone for the amniocentesis test in the private health care and she found that it is male baby. She became pregnant and delivered a male child. When the child grew older, he developed lumps in both his hands. She consulted so many doctors, but could not get the satisfactory answer. At last, she went to AIIMS, Delhi, for the consultation. After taking the detail history and diagnosis of his son, they could establish the fact that lumps are developed because of the fluid which was used at the time of performing amniocentesis test. Similar types of problem are also encountered by the other children whose mothers went for the same type of test. Thus, in doctor's opinion and in her belief it is side effect of the fluid which has been used for the test. Now, the child has grown and he has become young and of marriageable age, he is facing a lot of problem for finding a girl. The parents and prospective girls after knowing this problem are not ready to marry him. Thus, this younger boy is facing physical as well as social problems. He often asks her mother, why you have done this wrong to me? However, she cogently replies that it is the doctor who did not tell me the risk of the amniocentesis test and doctor has made me the guinea pig for their end.

Another woman recalled her amniocentesis test as a nurse giving local anesthesia and a doctor inserting a needle through the abdomen. Ultrasound monitoring during the piercing of the amniotic sac was not followed. The doctor used a stethoscope to locate the position of foetus. She believed that the needle was inserted many times because the doctor was unable to get the fluid. During the test, the doctor had mentioned repeatedly that there were no side effects. When finished, the nurse gave her the fluid to take to a diagnostic centre for testing, which she did before going home. The woman did not know that she had faced risks of miscarriage or premature labour because amniocentesis was used without the use of ultrasound; accidental injury inflicted on the foetus by the syringe is generally responsible for such risks. She was also unaware that such procedure might have led to sepsis in the reproductive tract.

The amniocentesis tests that are primarily meant to monitor the health of the child in the womb are not done; rather, they are used as a tool for female foeticide. In some cases where such tests are used for monitoring the health of the child, they are also carelessly used, which has resulted in the abnormalities of the children born and has also caused reproductive problems in women.

WOMEN AND BREASTFEEDING

Breastfeeding offers health as well as emotional benefits to infants and mothers. The baby gets protected against allergies; bonding between mother and child contributes to reduction in postpartum depression and gives mother a rest from the reproductive cycle through lactational amenorrhoea, which has many benefits: no anaemia, fatigue, protects against breast cancer, makes baby feel secure and gives the baby the safest and the perfect food for complete development.

Despite being known as a breastfeeding nation, India had to enact the Infant Milk Substitute (IMS) Act in 1992 to protect breastfeeding from the commercial onslaught of companies out to make a profit at the expense of the health of infants. The Act was later amended in 2003 and came into force on 1 January 2004. The main reason that more and more mothers are turning to infant formulas is because companies selling infant food make them psychological prisoners to the belief that their product is superior to mother's milk and thus more healthy for their newborn, although the contrary is true. Any such propaganda or advertisement or allurement to doctors or medical staff is a criminal offence and is punishable under the Act.

The National Family Health Survey (NFHS-3), published in 2007, stated that only 24.5 per cent of new mothers initiated breastfeeding in the hour after birth, 46.4 per cent breastfed exclusively the first six months and a slightly more encouraging 56.7 per cent nursed beyond six months with the introduction of complementary food.

But underweight was observed in nearly half of the children who were under the age of five years. The survey mentions these numbers in the same breath as a 57 in 1,000 live birth infant mortality rate (IMR) compared to 44 in 1,000 live births of sub-Saharan Africa. An important developmental parameter, IMR continues to stay high despite the two-decade-long campaign to bring it down. Breastfeeding promotion alone contributes to 11.6 per cent reduction in IMR if coverage of promotion is 99 per cent through one-to-one and group counselling, and can avert 21.9 million disability-adjusted life years at three years. With such staggering statistics lined up, the country needs to give breastfeeding an impetus. The solution is simple: promote breastfeeding by committing money and resources (NFHS-3, 2007). The NFHS-I in Kerala reported that 49 per cent of mothers had squeezed the first breast milk (N = 1423). This indicates that the governmental policy has partially helped, and many still continue to avoid giving first milk to their babies.

An International Working Group on infant feeding convened by the WHO (1991) recommended exclusive breastfeeding up to the first four months. Exclusive breastfeeding indicates feeding a baby with only breast milk and not with any supplementary foods (Ebrahim, 1978).

UNENFORCED LAW AND MISINFORMATION

A study done by Breastfeeding Promotion Network of India (BPNI), headquartered in New Delhi, suggests that the main stumbling block is the lack of support for mothers from the family, society, medical fraternity and also their work places. Mothers are often asked to throw away immune-property-rich colostrums or the first milk. Older women in the family, who dictate infant feeding practices for new mothers, cite inadequate breast milk supply and encourage mothers to switch to infant milk substitutes. Coupled with the aggressive promotion of these substitutes through surrogate advertisements, breastfeeding rates continue to be low. Surprisingly, it is not the law that is deficient, but instead its implementation and formation of support structure.

The Infant Milk Substitute, Feeding Bottles and Infant Food (Regulation of Production, Supply and Distribution) Act of 1992 does not ban the products under its scope, regulates marketing of breast milk substitutes, which the Act calls infant milk substitutes, to children under the age of two years, clearly in consonance with the World Health Organization recommendation of breastfeeding till two years. The IMS Act aims at curtailing misinformation and misdirected education of pregnant women and mothers of infants about breastfeeding, and prohibiting contact between industry and pregnant women or mothers of infants. Instead of just regulating the baby food industry, the Act also mandates creating awareness among pregnant women and lactating mothers about the benefits of breastfeeding. When read with other laws such as the Maternity Benefit Act, the law could adequately serve to increase breastfeeding.

Apart from benefits to the mother and child, economic value of breastfeeding is quite high. According to 1998 Breastfeeding Promotion Network of India (BPNI) estimate, the value of breast milk and breastfeeding to this country of 24.4 million annual births, based on the national breastfeeding patterns over a two-year lactation period, was around three times the national education budget then. Little wonder then that the manufacturers of infant milk substitutes have been trying to subvert the IMS Act. Surrogate advertising and sponsored medical conferences were the norm till BPNI took on food products major, Nestle, in 1994. Nestle products such as Cerelac and Lactogen were found to be violating provisions for advertising, labelling and sponsoring medical events. In the face of strong lobby, the government has failed to meet the targets and had set itself for the Tenth Five-Year Plan ending 2007 vis-à-vis breastfeeding (50 per cent initiating breastfeeding, 70 per cent exclusive breastfeeding for six months and 75 per cent complementary foods with breastfeeding until two years). And to the activists in BPNI, it is clearly the case of lack of information, support, lack of skills among health workers in an institutional delivery and finally social taboos devaluing breastfeeding.

The women on whom we focused our interview reported that as and when they complained of 'not enough milk', they are usually asked to buy formula milk or top feeding rather than making efforts for breast milk. In the Indian Medical Service, the Infant Milk Substitutes, Feeding Bottles and Infant Foods (Regulation of Production, Supply and Distribution) Act of 1992 mentions that:

> Inappropriate feeding practices lead to infant malnutrition, morbidity and infant milk substitutes and related products like feeding bottles and teats do constitute a health hazard. Promotions of infant milk substitutes and related products have been more extensive and pervasive

than the dissemination of information concerning the advantages of mother's milk and breastfeeding and contributes to decline in breastfeeding (IMS Act, 1992).

One of the women in our study reported that she was not taught how to breastfeed in the hospital and she explained her situation:

> I delivered a child in the hospital. When I complained to the hospital staff for not enough milk, the hospital staff did not make efforts to help for getting milk through breast. Thus, my child remained deprived of breastfeeding.

> Another woman said that since she and her baby were exposed to pain killers at birth, therefore, the feeding did not start immediately. To compensate the feeding of child she was encouraged for the formula milk. In the meantime the child and mother both felt comfortable with bottle feeding. Thus, breastfeeding was discouraged. Thus, it resulted into encouragement to bottlefeed instead of breastfeed.

Lack of information and support from the family also deprive women and children in terms of health as one woman observed:

> I had C-sections delivery and therefore, the breastfeeding did not start immediately. When I returned home, I was again exposed to more taboos and misinformation and therefore, the breast feeding did not take place.

WORKING MOTHERS AND BREASTFEEDING

Agriculture taking a backseat and growing urbanization has meant that most of the efforts of health workers get diluted. Daily wage earners, be it agricultural labourers or construction workers, traditionally used to take their children to workplace and breastfeed on demand. Increasing contractualization of labour has meant employment practices that are not mother- and child-friendly. The woman said:

> My nutritionally rich breast milk goes waste because I have to return to work to supplement family income. My employer forbids me to take nursing breaks or bringing my infant to the work site. Thus, I abandoned breastfeeding.

This phenomenon is equally seen in urban organized sectors. Employers, be it the state or private institutions, often do not offer a maternity leave with benefits in excess of the minimum six weeks prescribed under the Maternity Benefits Act 1961. Although the maternity leave available under this law varies from state to state, with Haryana and Punjab providing for six months, others such as Tamil Nadu give 135 days or three months' leave. There is a long-standing demand that the Act be amended to extend the minimum leave to six months and implement it uniformly across the country.

However, the lack of a policy framework to promote breastfeeding, the powerful supplementary foods lobby and the lack of support for mothers and health workers under-prepared in human lactation have meant that the seven-day-long push loses steam as the year rolls around. Breastfeeding and its success depend on hormonal control, particularly the flow of the mother's milk, which depends on her state of mind. If there is any doubt planted in her mind about her ability to lactate, it is unlikely that she will succeed. Therefore, health workers or care providers have to play a vital role in building up the confidence of new mothers. However, such support is rarely forthcoming. If a woman complains of 'not enough milk', she is usually asked to buy a formula feed rather than helping her gain confidence (Gupta, 2008).

WOMEN AND ABORTION

Some 42 million unintended pregnancies are terminated each year, an estimated 20 million of which are unsafe; two-thirds of all unsafe abortions occur among women aged between 15 and 30 years. Unsafe abortions kill an estimated 65,000–70,000 women every year, representing 13 per cent as all pregnancy-related deaths. In addition, they are associated with considerable morbidity; for instance, more than 3 million suffer from the effects of reproductive infection, and almost 1.7 million will develop secondary infertility (WHO, 2007).

Abortion has been legal in India since 1972, when the Medical Termination of Pregnancy (MTP) Act was passed. Under the Act, abortion is legal if it endangers the life of the woman or causes grave injury to her physical or mental health, or is likely to result in the birth of a baby with physical or mental abnormalities or is a result of rape or contraceptive failure. The Act further stated that abortions could take place in government-approved health facilities specifically approved for conducting abortions and by registered medical practitioner.

Data providing consistent estimates of induced abortion in India are scarce: whatever is available is through government reports and surveys. Available abortion statistics shows that 5–6 million abortions occur in unapproved facilities (Ganatra, 2000; Arnold et al., 2002).

Illegal abortions are 8–11 times as high as legal abortions (Chhabra and Nuna, 1994; Jessani and Iyer, 1995; Chhabra, 1996).

In the MTP Act, it is the medical doctor who decides whether an abortion seeker fulfils the criteria spelled out in the Act. It is the doctor who decides as to how liberally or restrictively to interpret the Act in a given socio-political context. In addition to other factors, providers' attitude towards and understanding of women and their abortion needs, influence the interpretation of the Act, which is an important variable influencing women's access to abortion services. Bandewar (2003) finds that the pattern of abortion practice indicates that perceptions and concerns for women's health in the context of their abortion needs do not go with their abortion care service pattern. This is because a large number of providers have mentioned that it was not advisable for women to use abortion as spacing method. One expects that they would provide contraceptive counselling to women seeking abortion care to avoid repetitive abortions. Contraceptives were forced without leaving much space for making informed choices and denying opportunities to educate themselves vis-à-vis contraceptives.

One woman reports:

> When I became pregnant for the third time I decided to go for abortion. I with a neighbour went to civil hospital. The lady doctor agreed for abortion but said that I must accept sterilization also. I became very much nervous. I did not want to go through operation and hence came back.

The women in our study had incorrect knowledge of the legality of abortion. They said that abortions among widows and unmarried girls are illegal. Some women had a more nuanced understanding of the abortion legislation in India; they explained that all abortions performed in private facilities or beyond 14 weeks' gestation are illegal. These women also believed that husband's consent is required by law before abortion can take place. One woman observed and said that doctors have a different opinion about the legality of the abortion:

> One of the doctors said that just because abortion is legalized, does not mean that doctors should be so liberal in doing this.

The Mumbai High Court judgement disallowing the abortion of a 26-week-old foetus has sparked off a nationwide debate on abortion and a woman's right of choice. But for a majority of Indian women, MTP remains largely unsafe (*The Times of India*, 2008).

UNSAFE AND INADEQUATE NUMBER OF ABORTION FACILITIES

Unsafe abortions are those performed illegally by untrained practitioners with faulty equipment, leading to injuries, infections and even death. India has the highest number of unsafe abortions in the world. According to government estimates, 8.9 per cent of maternal deaths in India every year—around 15,000—are caused by unsafe abortions. The irony is apparent when doctors say MTP, if done right, is among the safest medical procedures. Of the 6.4 million abortions performed in India in 2002 and 2003, 56 per cent or 3.6 million were unsafe, says the Abortion Assessment Project I, 2004. The study—one of the largest in recent times—was managed by the Mumbai-based Centre for Equity into Health and Allied Themes and Healthwatch Trust. It included qualitative and quantitative studies across various states by non-governmental organizations (NGOs), researchers and healthcare professionals (Duggal and Ramachandran, 2004).

'There's inadequate, inequitable distribution of facilities for safe abortions. Contraceptive usage is low in India, hence the great demand for safe abortion services', said Dr Jaydeep Tank, Chairperson of the MTP Committee at the Federation of Obstetric and Gynaecological Societies of India (FOGSI). Besides, only 6 per cent of India's 23,000 Primary Health Centres provide abortion services. 'Besides risk to life, unsafe abortions have serious long-term repercussions like lifelong disabilities and reproductive tract infections', said Sushanta Banerjee, senior advisor at Ipas, an NGO (*The Times of India*, 2008).

ABORTION LAWS

For a country with a 'liberal' law on abortion, Banerjee said awareness about it is extremely low even three decades after it was enacted. 'In Jharkhand, for instance, we found that 82 per cent of women didn't even know abortion was legal', he said. In a related study by the Population Council in Rajasthan in 2002, the figure was 84 per cent and in Maharashtra at least 37 per cent of those who had had abortions thought they were illegal. This misconception leads many women to unqualified professionals. Other barriers to safe abortion are 'social stigma and myths attached to MTP', said Tank. 'Awareness about abortion through drugs like Mifepristone and Misoprostol is also low, despite they being legal and easily available' (Elul et al., 2004).

Social barriers such as spousal consent and judgemental doctors are also deterrents, though the law requires no such consent. Under the government's Reproductive and Child Health Project, safe abortions are a key concern and some progress is being made—maternal mortality due to abortion was 11 per cent in 2001. 'We need to generate awareness at the community level about contraception and safe abortion, in both rural areas and urban slums', said Thomas Chandy, CEO, Save The Children in India. Ipas also advocates training of mid-level service providers such as nurses and non-allopathic doctors in remote areas where access to trained doctors is a problem (*The Times of India*, 2008).

Abortion remains highly restricted, and unsafe abortion is common and continues to damage women's health. The evidence is strong that empowering women with the means to decide for themselves when to become pregnant and how many children to have significantly lowers unintended pregnancy rates and thereby reduces the need for abortion. One woman had gone to the family planning centre for abortion and she shared her experience with us:

> I went for the MTP to the government facility they agreed for the MTP but without going for contraceptive in the form of 'Copper-T' I cannot leave the hospital. Secondly, since I was in my early twenties therefore, they asked me to bring accompanied person, either husband or some-one else.

Another woman reported:

> I went to the family planning clinic for the MTP. But the doctor was not ready to do MTP as he was telling other health personnel that these women do not come for contraceptive advice and even if they come it is very difficult to convince them about family planning. Most women come here to get rid of pregnancies through MTP. They never plan pregnancies. These types of accusation are made against us. Thus I feel that the MTP is done with negative attitude to make me realize that I have committed a crime and therefore, I am guilty of the same.

ACCESS TO POST-ABORTION CARE

The mortality rates and severity of short- or long-term complications of unsafe abortions may be strongly influenced by the quality of care received after the abortion. Acute complications such as uterine perforation or the perforation or injury of other internal organs may be fatal if emergency care is not urgently provided. Infection will progress locally and systematically as long as the proper medical and surgical therapy is not given. The later and the less efficient the care received, the more severe the consequences are likely to be and the greater the risk of death. Therefore, it is recommended that the assessment of the woman's condition and the provision of post-abortion should be available on a 24-hour basis and provided with the urgency demanded by the severity of the condition (Look, 2011).

It also pointed out the problems of reach and access with public investment in abortion facilities being woefully inadequate. Only 25 per cent of abortion facilities in the organized sector are government-owned; the rest are private clinics. These are so expensive that they completely exclude the poor sections.

In one of the study, Das et al. (2004) found that MTP was done also with laparoscopic legations, in contravention to medical standards. A bicycle pump with a nasal tube attached to its end was used to pump air into the abdomen; and in some cases, the bulb of a blood pressure instrument was used to pump air. Carbon dioxide was not at all used.

In India, abortion is regulated on grounds of the health of the mother. It has since been widely interpreted in practice to mean that the health of the mother would suffer from too many pregnancies. Abortion is widely used as a contraceptive measure by women. Further, the sex-selective abortion on non-medical grounds brought out the difficulty with the slogan 'a woman's right to choose'. It threw up a new dilemma: Can the right of women to decide regarding abortion be extended to women's use of prenatal diagnosis and abortion of a female foetus? Most Indian feminists, while supporting women's rights to abortion, condemned the practice of sex-selective abortion and succeeded in having it banned in 1994 (Gupta, 2000: 602). The field data confirm that respondents were rarely aware of the legality of abortion.

CONCLUSION

The paper is divided into three main parts. The first part reflects on the understanding of women and their health rights. The second part, which is empirical in nature and based on the narratives of women, discerns the nature of health complications and procedures with family planning, amniocentesis test, breastfeeding and abortion. It also analyses the conflicting situation arising out of the women's health rights issues. The third part concludes by problematizing the autonomy and right of the women in the above context. The women need urgent attention in the broader context of individual freedom and human ethics.

REFERENCES

Arnold, F., S. Kishor and T.K. Roy, 2002, 'Sex-Selective Abortions in India', *Population and Development Review*, 28(4): 759–85.

Balasurbrahmanyan, V., 1986, *Contraception: As if Women Mattered: A Critique of Family Planning*. Bombay: Centre for Education and Documentation.

Bandewar, Sunita, 2003, 'Abortion Services and Providers' Perceptions: Gender Dimensions', *Economic and Political Weekly*, XXXVIII(21): 2081.

Chhabra, R., 1996, 'Abortion in India: An Overview', *Demography India*, 25(1): 83–92.

Chhabra, R. and S.C. Nuna, 1994, *Abortion in India: An Overview*. New Delhi: Ford Foundation.

Das, Abhijit, Ramkant Rai and Dinesh Singh, 2004, 'Medical Negligence and Rights Violation', *Economic and Political Weekly*, August 28–September 3, 39(35): 3876–79.

Duggal, Ravi and Vimla Ramachandran, 2004, 'The Abortion Assessment Project- India: Key Findings and Recommendations', *Reproductive Health Matters* (Supplement), 12(24): 122–29.

Ebrahim, G.J., 1978, *Breastfeeding- The Biological Option, Macmillan Tropical Community Health Manuals*. London: Macmillan Press.

Elul, Batya, Sandhya Barge, Shalini Verma, Rajani Ved, Rajesh Singh and Karin Lockwood, 2004, *Unwanted Pregnancy and Induced Abortion in Rajasthan, India: A Qualitative Exploration*. New Delhi: Population Council and Ibtada.

Ganatra, B.R., 2000, 'Abortion Research in India: What We Know, and What We Need to Know'. In *Women's Reproductive Health in India*, edited by Radhika Ramasubban and Shireen J. Jejeebhoy, New Delhi: Rawat Publications.

Gupta, Arun, 2008, 'Manipulation by Assistance: Undermining Breastfeeding', *Economic and Political Weekly*, September 6, XLIII(36).

Gupta, Jyotsna Agnihotri, 2000, *New Reproductive Technologies, Women's health and Autonomy*. New Delhi: Sage Publications.

IMS Act, 1992, *Infant Milk Substitutes, Feeding Bottle and Infant Foods (Regulation of Production, Supply and Distribution)* Act No. 41 of 1992, Government of India, Ministry of Law, Justice and Company Affairs, 29 December 1992.

International Institute of Population Sciences (IIPS) and Macro International, 2007, *National Family Health Survey (NFHS-3) 2005–06, India: Key Findings*. Mumbai: IIPS.

Jessani, A. and A. Iyer, 1995, 'Abortions: Who is Responsible for Her Rights?' In *Our Lives our Health*, edited by Malini Karkal, New Delhi: Coordination Unit, The World Conference on Women, Beijing.

Karkal, Malini, 1985, 'Maternal and Infant Mortality', *Economic and Political Weekly*, 20(43): 1835–37.

Look, Paul E.A. Van, 2011, *Sexual and Reproductive Health: A Public Health Perspective*. The Netherlands: Elsevier.

Mavalankar, D. and Bharti Sharma, 1999, 'The Quality of Care in Sterilization Camp: Evidence from Gujarat'. In *Improving Quality of Care in India's Family Welfare Programme*, edited by M.A. Koenig and M.E. Khan, New York: Population Council.

Nagla, Madhu, 2007, 'Health and Culture: An Interface'. In *Health Dynamics and Marginalized Communities*, edited by Mohammad Akram, Jaipur: Rawat Publications.

Prakash, P., 1984, 'Use of Laparoscopy for Sterilizations', *Economic and Political Weekly*, March 17: 453–54.

Rajya Sabha, 2003, *Unstarred Question No. 752*, answered on 28 July 2003.

Ram, K., 1998, 'Maternity and the Story of Enlightenment in the Colonies: Tamilnadu Women, South India'. In *Maternities and Modernities in Colonial and Post Colonial Experiences in Asia and the Pacific*, edited by K. Ram and M. Jolly, Cambridge: Cambridge University Press, pp. 114–43.

Ramanathan, M., R. Dilip and S.S. Padmadas, 1995, 'Quality of Care in Laparoscopic Sterilization Camps: Observations from Kerala, India', *Reproductive Health Matters*, 6 (November): 84–93.

The Times of India, 2008, *Most Unsafe Abortions in India*, August 9.

The Times of India, 2012, *53 Women Sterilized in Bihar in 2 Hours*, April 3.

Unnithan-Kumar, Maya, 2003, 'Spirits of the Womb: Migration, Reproductive Choice and Healing in Rajasthan', *Contribution to Indian Sociology*, 37 (1–3): 184.

WHO, 1991, *Indicators for Assessing Breast-Feeding Practices*, Report on an Informal Meeting, June 11–12. Geneva: WHO.

WHO, 2007, *Unsafe Abortion: Global and Regional Estimates of Incidence of Unsafe Abortion and Associated Mortality in 2000*. Geneva: WHO.

CHAPTER 3

Social Determinants of Maternal and Child Health in India: Macro–Micro Disjunctions

K.R. Nayar and Lekha Bhat

Persistently high maternal mortality ratio (MMR) is one of the most worrisome problems plaguing the Indian Health Service. There are several interventions currently in place to bring down the high MMR. Some of the important health system interventions related to maternal health have larger sociological than biomedical dimensions. The Janani Suraksha Yojana (JSY), which offers conditional cash transfer to women for institutional deliveries, and the use of Accredited Social Health Activists (ASHAs) are supposed to take care of the high out-of-pocket expenditure, the consequent impoverishment due to accessing health care and the social exclusion and lack of access to health care. The programme is also intended to reduce home deliveries that are assumed to be one of the reasons for the high mortality of mothers. However, the central issues with respect to institutional deliveries from a sociological point of view are social exclusion and inequalities in maternal care and the issue of social dignity when women utilize institutions for birthing. This chapter examines social dimensions such as social exclusion and dignity with respect to maternal health and maternal health care using macro- and micro-data and demonstrates the disjunctions with macro- and micro-data with respect to outcomes of the programmes initiated in recent times.

SOCIAL EXCLUSION AND MATERNAL HEALTH

One of the important social determinants that need to be addressed with respect to the Indian Health Service system is 'social exclusion'. Social exclusion, as conceptualized by many scholars such as Amartya Sen, mainly refers to the inability of our society to keep all groups and individuals within reach of what we expect as society to realize their full potential. Marginalization of certain groups or classes occurs in most societies including developed countries, and perhaps it is more pronounced in underdeveloped countries. Economic capability (poverty), gender, age, caste and religion, etc., are important variables that indicate exclusion from social and economic opportunities. In the Indian context, caste may be considered the most important indicator of social exclusion and broadly as a proxy for socio-economic status and poverty. In the identification of the poor, scheduled castes and scheduled tribes and in some cases the other backward castes are considered socially disadvantaged groups, and such groups have a higher probability of living under adverse conditions and poverty. The health status and utilization patterns of such groups give an indication of their social exclusion as well as an idea of the linkages between poverty and health. Data on utilization of antenatal care (ANC) among different caste groups in India which are based on the National Family Health Survey-2, highlight the caste differentials in health (Table 3.1). The proportion of scheduled caste and scheduled tribe women who have not availed any antenatal care is considerably higher compared to other castes. The difference is most glaring at higher level of care such as from doctors.

On the whole, the data available suggest that the marginalized sections such as scheduled castes/scheduled tribes and other backward castes who are also poor in India suffer from a 'social gap' in terms of health status and health services. Specific behavioural practices in childbirth or early child development are closely linked to the social and cultural background of the population. It is now well known that behavioural practices including health actions are rooted in the social, political and cultural context. However, the specific pathways of such social variables and health are not well researched, which often results in half-baked and unifocused actions such as behavioural change programmes or educational activities. What is required is a more multi-focused action on vulnerable sections of the population, which can, not only take care of the specific social vulnerabilities

Table 3.1 Percentage of Utilization of Antenatal Care by Social Groups in India

Sources of antenatal care	*Social groups*	*NFHS-1 (1992–93)*	*NFHS-2 (1998–99)*	*NFHS-3 (2005–06)*
ANC at home by health workers	SC	14.6	5.9	NA
	ST	18.5	10.0	NA
	OBC	NA	5.9	NA
	Others	11.9	4.0	NA
Doctors	SC	29.4	41.7	42.0
	ST	21.0	34.7	32.8
	OBC	NA	48.9	48.4
	Others	44.0	56.5	63.6
Other health professionals	SC	12.8	13.3	0.7
	ST	7.1	11.5	1.0
	OBC	NA	9.6	0.8
	Others	9.1	10.6	1.6
Traditional birth attendants and others	SC	0.2	0.2	1.5
	ST	0.2	0.3	2.3
	OBC	NA	0.2	0.7
	Others	0.3	0.2	1.1
No ANC	SC	42.2	38.2	25.9
	ST	52.3	43.1	29.4
	OBC	NA	34.8	25.5
	Others	34.0	27.9	15.2

Source: International Institute for Population Sciences (1995, 2007); International Institute for Population Sciences and ORC Macro (2000).

NA, not available.

such as unemployment, social exclusion, etc., but can also enhance accessibility and availability of health services. Health service system should take into cognizance such issues to be able to achieve universal health care. The goals of achieving reductions in mortality rate under five and the maternal mortality rate by two-thirds (fourth and fifth Millennium Development Goals or MDGs) are also contingent upon addressing some of these important social determinants.

Among the different packages that the National Rural Health Mission (NRHM) flagged, the JSY is claimed to have made some impact on institutional deliveries. The JSY programme is an effort to bring the poor, excluded and marginalized women closer to the health services system through a facilitatory and participatory approach with the objective of reducing maternal and neonatal mortality. The ASHAs who are women from the same community under this programme serve as the link to motivate and support the women. The JSY is a programme that combines economic support and facilitatory approaches to enhance institutional deliveries in rural areas. Public health scholars have raised a number of issues with regard to the JSY. One controversy is with regard to the overemphasis on institutional deliveries given the long-term mistrust of government health services, that is, the credibility gap and the caste, class and gender bias when women access care (Jeffrey and Jeffrey, 2010). The second issue is with regard to the component of privatization, which some public health scholars argue could lead to further weakening of public sector health services (Nayar, 1998). Many states have started contracting private sector doctors and private hospitals for increasing the number of institutional deliveries. The third issue is with regard to the approach of conditional cash transfer and the argument is difficult to attribute cash transfer alone to positive outcomes (Lagarde et al., 2009). Despite such critiques, some states in India have introduced people-friendly and socially and culturally oriented innovations in the JSY programme, although these could be in the form of small steps.

The impacts of these initiatives are not measurable yet. But as evident from the responses of grass-roots-level workers, there are shifts in the way in which the health services are perceived by the people. Availability of services has changed the negative perceptions of public sector services. Study findings indicate a huge increase in the utilization of the JSY scheme. In order to reach the stated goal of 80 per cent institutional deliveries, more capacity needs to be created in health systems to cater to this JSY-induced demand (UNICEF, 2009; Government of India, 2011). Methodologically, it is necessary to state that the impact of the policy initiatives on addressing inclusion has to be seen in deductive terms. The measurable change is in terms of health indices, that is, reduction in maternal mortality rate and infant mortality rate. However, it is possible to assume that such changes are due to the policy and programme shifts focusing on the women below the poverty line who, by and large, belong to the underprivileged castes in India. Moreover, the strong linkage between such focused action and the reduction in inequity is evident from a larger share of JSY beneficiaries among women who access facility-based care for deliveries. This is found out by both the Common Review Mission and the United National Population Fund (UNFPA)'s Concurrent Assessment.

The UNFPA (2009) evaluation conducted in five states revealed considerable improvement in institutional deliveries (Figure 3.1). Madhya Pradesh and Rajasthan, which belong to the vulnerable states, have recorded high institutional deliveries when compared to the previous years. Although such a trend has not led to dramatic decline of MMR as reflected from the MMR figures released in 2011, the decline for the vulnerable states has been from 375 in 2004–06 to 308 in 2007–09: a decline of about 18 per cent, which can be called as 'significant' (see also Figure 3.2). The all-India figure shows that MMR declined from 254 in 2004–06 to 202 in 2007–09: a fall of about 17 per cent. Apart from Kerala, Tamil Nadu and Maharashtra have also joined the states that achieved the MDG target (Government of India: http://censusindia.gov.in/vital_statistics/SRS_Bulletins/Bulletins.aspx; see Figure 3.2 for some selected states). Kerala witnessed dramatic increase in institutional deliveries, which went up from 87.8 per cent in 1992–93 to 99.5 per cent in 2004–05. However, the linkage between high rates of institutional deliveries and MMR reductions is yet to be empirically demonstrated, and the associations are based on the evidence from Kerala.

District Level Household Survey (DLHS) 2 and 3 data from 2002–04 and 2007–08 show that Odisha and West Bengal are the two states that have recorded considerable improvement with respect to antenatal check-up across different caste groups. Not only is there improvement in the figures in these two states, but the social gap between different caste groups has also reduced. However, in most other states, the effect of antenatal coverage was smaller. Other

Figure 3.1 Institutional Deliveries in Rural Areas of Selected States of India 1998–08

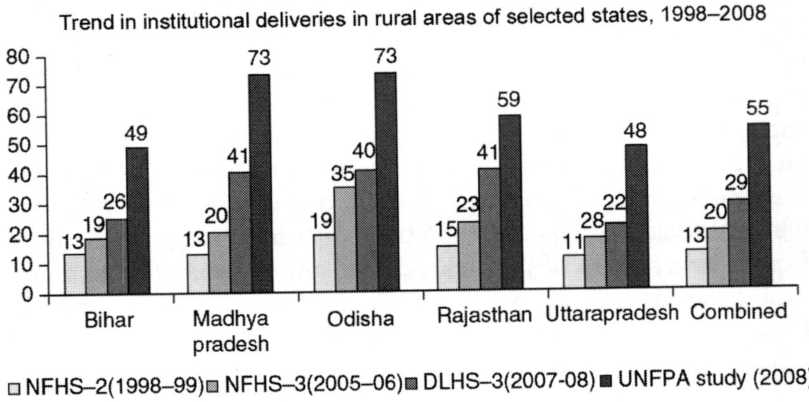

Source: UNFPA, 2009.

Figure 3.2 Maternal Mortality Rates in Selected States 2004 and 2007

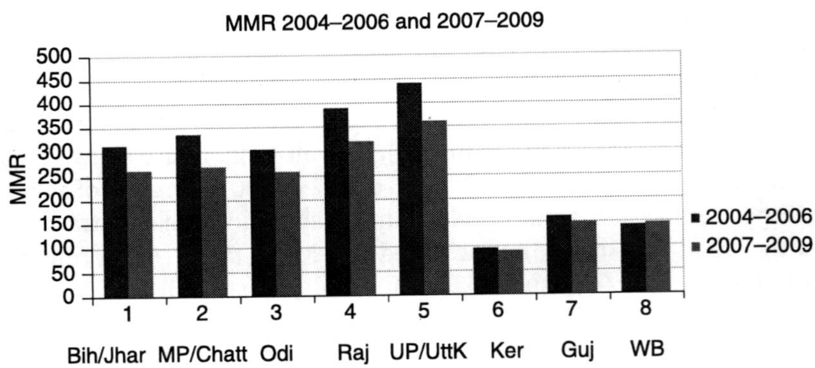

Source: Registrar General of India, *Special Bulletin on Maternal Mortality in India 2004–06 and 2007–09*, April 2009 and June 2011.

analyses based on NFHS rounds, and DLHS also show that the states have moved to higher equity with respect to institutional deliveries (Shekhar and Ram, 2011). The linkage between cash assistance and increase in institutional care is evident from the increase in institutional deliveries especially in high-focus states such as Madhya Pradesh although this increase could be highly skewed and localized which is not reflected in the aggregate data. Preliminary analysis based on DLHS data shows that the JSY scheme has helped in the coverage of antenatal and intrapartum care and has also probably contributed to reductions in the numbers of perinatal and neonatal deaths, although the effect on maternal mortality is not known (Lim et al., 2010). The uptake of JSY among the poorest and least educated women has also not been high. The explanations for this trend are (1) short duration of the JSY scheme, (2) problems in the physical access and (3) cultural barriers against institutional births among certain groups (Lim et al., 2010). DLHS data also show that with respect to immunization coverage, there is considerable improvement in states such as Odisha, West Bengal, Chhattisgarh and Uttarakhand, especially among the SC/ST communities. The issue of whether the JSY could reduce inequities in care is still an open question that needs further investigation (Das et al., 2011). For the moment, it is a matter of deduction that because coverage has increased as evident from the data, the programme could have led to some spin-offs on increasing access and acceptability of health services among the underprivileged sections in the country.

It is however necessary to examine whether such quantitative increase in utilization has led to well-being of women who seek care especially in terms of actual reductions in exclusion and improvements in terms of dignity of birthing. This is attempted in the following section through an inductive process attempted in two public hospitals as part of a larger study to understand the processes and the context in which human dignity is violated in maternity wards of public hospitals in Kerala. The fieldwork over a period of three months included ward visits, observing childbirth in the birthing room and house visits.

DIGNITY AND INCLUSION/EXCLUSION IN INSTITUTIONAL CHILDBIRTH

Institutional deliveries have become medicalized and commercialized to the extent that women are not actively engaged with their birthing experience, but they are mere recipients of the services. In this process, a woman's dignity is encountered/dishonoured. The concept of dignity assumes centre stage because encounters on human dignity are persistent events that have severe negative impacts on an individual's social well-being and self-identity.[1] Scholarly literature has not focused much on the violation of dignity and exclusion that are taking place while women utilize institutions for their birthing needs.

Social Dignity and Institutional Childbirth

At the time of fieldwork, we could observe rampant violations of women's dignity during childbirth. Nurses and other paramedical staff would shout loudly and rudely at the birthing women. The birthing women never dared to ask any questions nor attempted to clarify their doubts. These shouting scenes were more common if the birthing women reached the hospital during night shift hours. The body language shown was that of rejection and contempt.

Women felt that the practice of using caste/religious names and numbers to identify them threaten one's self-identity and increased the feelings of exclusion. They were addressed as 'primy in third bed', 'Nair woman who is in left extreme', etc. Muslim women were especially marked and insults being thrown at them. Further, it was observed that nurses in their private talk use caste names to identify the women. Upper-caste names were used as suffix (e.g. Ms X. Nair), whereas lower-caste names along with other insulting names were thrown at liberally for the *Pulaya* community[2] who screamed and cried loudly during birthing.

Another aspect that the women informants highlighted was the tendency of the hospital staff to use sexually vulgar comments and veiled threats. Because of pain, anxiety and helplessness, birthing women did not reply. They feared that, if they replied, the existing level of care they were getting (after scolding, shouting and screaming) would be withheld and that survival of the baby would be threatened.

The women respondents shared their experiences of physical violence and torture. This included slapping, pinching on the thighs, hair pulling, etc. The respondents considered this as humiliation where they were not given minimal recognition as human beings. The respondents felt that the complexion of one's body, dressing style and clothes provoked the health care providers to consider that some women were not very serious about having a safe childbirth. Women who belonged to scheduled caste/Muslim community reported more incidences of physical violence.

Women who belonged to Muslim community felt that they were mostly considered 'study cases' for the trainee MBBS students. Such objectification and experimentation on their bodies without their consent was an affront to women's dignity. On clarification, the doctors explained that Muslim women having had more number of children and thus having undergone more labour pain were suitable case studies on childbirth.

Women also believed that untouchability is practised covertly and implicitly in the hospitals. The women who were darker, having marks on their face and thighs, etc., were considered unclean and irresponsible. Scheduled caste women felt that doctors were not examining them thoroughly.

It was also observed that health care providers did not prefer to share information with the birthing women. The respondents mentioned that their dignity was affected because they were considered 'illiterates who do not know anything about pregnancy/ childbirth'. Information such as birth weight of the foetus, progress in labour, etc., was of utmost importance to them, as it would help them remain active throughout the birthing process and boost their confidence. In the birthing room, the birthing tables were not separated using curtains, etc. Privacy and confidentiality was not maintained at any stage. When the birthing room was crowded, women were asked to share a common bed (before they were in the active stage of labour and were shifted to birthing tables).

The Context of Dignity Violation in Hospitals

The interaction between the birthing women and the health care providers is asymmetrical and hierarchical in nature. Women due to their lack of professional knowledge and physical condition (here, their pregnancy) are in a vulnerable position. Apart from this, the health care providers make constant and conscious attempts to exercise their power, which in turn would ensure their professional autonomy and supremacy. Medicalization and commercialization of childbirth are the ways in which medical supremacy is ensured in childbirth.

Medicalization and commercialization of childbirth are two aspects that are responsible for ensuring multiple levels of oppression and exploitation in the public hospitals. Childbirth has become intensely medicalized and a number of new technologies are adopted to assist the birthing women. The indiscriminate use of such technologies actually limits birthing women's freedom and makes them more dependent on the health care providers. Similarly, the introduction of user fee, corruption and bribery at public hospitals, etc., has led to a condition in which poor women are exploited.

In the public hospitals where the fieldwork was conducted, the expenses during childbirth varied from ₹ 5,000 to 12,000 although treatment is expected to be completely free of cost. Apart from this, JSY is expected to help the birthing women meet their out-of-pocket expenditure. But when birthing women are forced to pay bribes and other user charges, the schemes such as JSY become redundant and economic burden/debt of the family increases.

The lack of space, medical equipment and other medical/infrastructural/manpower resources is also an important factor to be considered. Lack of enough number of beds, crowded birthing room, etc., ensure that birthing women have negative and terrifying experience in the hospitals. Discrimination and exclusion occur when limited resources are divided among many, and one group is favoured over another based on caste/religion or on the ability to pay.

CONCLUDING OBSERVATIONS

From the data mentioned earlier, it is clear that not only access to maternal health care is more restricted for lower-caste people, but they are also subjected to more indignities at the hospital, leading to feelings of exclusion and alienation. The ability to pay (in terms of user fee/bribe/private consultation) determines the level of care and attention a birthing woman can receive. There exists long-term mistrust between birthing women and health care providers. Variables such as education of woman, caste, religion and socio-economic status also play an important role in determining the level of care that birthing women receive in the health care institutions.

The disjunction between macro- and micro-data is important from both a methodological and programme point of view. Methodologically, it shows the need for triangulation while reaching conclusions on programme effectiveness. The disjunctions between macro- and micro-data and deduction and induction could be explored further by undertaking studies in other states. Increasing institutional deliveries using conditional cash transfers or using other incentives through the JSY are important from the programme point of view. The sudden withdrawal of maternity services in vulnerable states leads us to assume that the social questions such as exclusion and marginalization have been addressed or the gap is narrowing.

However, micro-data from the state of Kerala, which is one of the better-performing states of India, show a picture that is contrary. The empirical observations demonstrate the vulnerabilities of women when they reach the institutions for birthing. The indignities that they go through and the exclusion and marginalization that they face are lessons worth considering for improving maternal health programmes.

NOTES

1. Human dignity does not distinguish between people and regardless of their social standing, it is shared by all (Pritchard, 1972). Schachter (1983) also gives an expression that dignity is about *worth*; it has links with self-respect and recognizes another individual's worth. Human dignity and social dignity also need to be distinguished here. Human dignity means a person's worth simply by virtue of being human. This focus on inherent worth of an individual is closely linked to the Kantian notion of human dignity to treat every human being as an end, not as a means. Individuals are not to be perceived or treated merely as instruments or objects of the will of others. Social dignity is that aspect which is developed in the interactions between individuals/collectives. Social dignity comprises the ways in which respect and worth is conveyed and reflected in the behaviour (Jacobson, 2009). It was human rights activist Mann (1998) who pioneered the idea of using the framework of dignity to explain the problems in public health. He opined that violation of dignity is a pathogenic force with a destructive capacity.
2. Scheduled caste in Kerala.

REFERENCES

Das, A., D. Rao and A. Hagopian, 2011, 'India's Janani Suraksha Yojana: Further Review Needed', *The Lancet*, 377: 295–96.

Government of India, *SRS Bulletins*, [online] available at http://censusindia.gov.in/vital_statistics/SRS_Bulletins/Bulletins.aspx (accessed on 4 March 2012).

Government of India, 2011, *Fourth Common Review Mission Report 2010*. New Delhi: NRHM, Ministry of Health and Family Welfare.

International Institute for Population Sciences, 1995, *National Family Health Survey (MCH and Family Planning), 1992–93, India*. Bombay: IIPS.

International Institute for Population Sciences, 2007, *National Family Health Survey (NFHS-3), 2004–05, Government of India*. Mumbai: IIPS.

International Institute for Population Sciences and ORC Macro, 2000, *National Family Health Survey (NFHS-2), 1998–99, Government of India*. Mumbai: IIPS.

Jacobson, N., 2009, 'Dignity Violation in Health Care', *Quality Health Research*, 19(11): 1536–47.

Jeffrey, P. and R. Jeffrey, 2010, 'Only When the Boat has Started Sinking: A Maternal Death in Rural North India', *Social Science and Medicine*, 71(10): 1711–18.

Lagarde, M., A. Haines and N. Palmer, 2009, 'The Impact of Conditional Cash Transfers on Health Outcomes and use of Health Services in Low and Middle Income Countries', *Cochrane Database of Systematic Reviews. Wiley Online Library*, [online] available at http://onlinelibrary.wiley.com/doi/10.1002/14651858.CD008137/abstract;jsessionid=E5D90E86904E4C7DA83D8406CC3C4A4F.d03t03 (accessed on 20 August 2011).

Lim, S.S., D. Lalit, J.A. Hoisington, S.L. James, M.C. Hogan and E. Gakidou, 2010, 'India's Janani Suraksha Yojana, a Conditional Transfer Programme to Increase Births in Health Facilities: An Impact Evaluation', *The Lancet*, 375: 2009–23.

Mann, J., 1998, 'Dignity and Health: The UDHR's Revolutionary First Article', *Health and Human Rights*, 3(2): 30–38.

Nayar, K.R., 1998, 'Old Priorities and New Agenda of Public Health in India: Is there a Mismatch?', *Croatian Medical Journal*, 39(3): 308–15.

Pritchard, M.S., 1972, 'Human Dignity and Justice', *Ethics*, 82(4): 299–313.

Registrar General of India, 2011, *Special Bulletin on Maternal Mortality in India 2007–09. Sample Registration System*. New Delhi: Government of India.

Schachter, O., 1983, 'Human Dignity as a Normative Concept', *The American Journal of International Law*, 77(4): 848–54.

Shekhar, C. and F. Ram, 2011, *In-Depth Analysis of Equity Differences in Health Outcomes Focusing on Reproductive and Child Health in Six Indian States*. Mumbai: IIPS.

UNFPA, 2009, *Concurrent Assessment of JSY in Selected States*. New Delhi: UNFPA.

UNICEF, 2009, *Coverage Evaluation Survey Report 2009*. New Delhi: UNICEF and Government of India.

CHAPTER 4

Do Women Benefit from Cancer Screening Programmes? Reflections from Fieldwork in Odisha

Suchitra Pradhan and Suhita Chopra Chatterjee

National Cancer Programmes worldwide rely heavily on screening for the early detection of breast and cervix cancer. However, in recent times, there have been polarized arguments about the benefits and harm of screening. This chapter looks into some of the ethical debates and questions the value of screening in India. Based on a study in Odisha, it identifies the structural and socio-economic barriers that make screening programmes lose their efficacy in India. In the light of the arguments presented, the chapter asks for a serious scientific rethinking of screening measures in order to save financial costs and redirect resources for evolving better treatment modalities.

Breast and cervix cancer are the leading cause of cancer-related mortality among women in India. Cancer of breast is expected to cross the figure of 100,000 by the year 2020. In the year 2010, around 68,903 cases of cervix cancer have been estimated to occur that may decrease to 53,654 cases by the year 2020 (Takiar et al., 2010).

The Indian scenario, more or less, replicates the pattern worldwide. But in developed countries despite increase in breast and cervical cancer, mortality over the past 25 years has been stable or decreasing. Such reductions have been attributed to screening, early detection and improved treatment. On the contrary, the disproportionate burden of deaths in developing countries and elsewhere in medically underserved populations is mainly due to the lack of screening and prevalence of unhygienic conditions. However, the benefit of screening as a public health measure is still debatable.

Most international experts argue that regular use of screening methods can detect cancers of the breast, colon, rectum, cervix and prostate at an early stage (Clasen et al., 1994) and that at least older women and those with a high-risk profile may gain additional years of life if their breast or genital cancer is detected and treated early (Fletcher et al., 1993; Kelsey and Bernstein, 1996; Shapiro et al., 1998). But there are researchers who have argued against the nature of screening programmes. According to Jepson et al. (2007), in screening for a particular condition, a large number of apparently healthy people are tested in order to identify a small number of people who have pre-clinical disease. Screening strategy works only when countries have a well-developed cancer screening programme, which includes an understanding of the natural history of the condition screened, existence of suitable tests that are acceptable to the population, agreed policy for diagnostic evaluation and effective treatment with evidence that it leads to better outcome (Wilson and Jungner, 1968; National Screening Committee-UK, 1998). The benefits of screening can be realized only when there is a follow-up of abnormal results and definitive testing is done (Mandelblatt et al., 1997). These conditions are rarely fulfilled by countries that conduct screening programmes. There is also considerable ambiguity about age-specific tests and the choice of screening tests, which best suits the needs of a particular country.

In the absence of necessary conditions, screening may bring about worry and anxiety among the target community. For those with a false-positive finding, preoccupation with symptoms and increased use of health services might last long past the reassuring diagnosis (Rimer and Bluman, 1997; Aro et al., 2000). A false-negative finding misleadingly reassures and delays diagnosis (Jepson et al., 2007). Further, Strong et al. (2005) stated that identification of either trivial or untreatable conditions can result in considerable waste of resources and anxiety with no practical outcome. Finding cancers that would never have become clinical in a lifetime is clearly a major adverse effect of screening (Irwig et al., 2006). Similarly, Marks et al. (2008) indicated that psychological distress to women and expenditure of screening in poor countries outweigh the benefits in terms of increased life expectancy. Rosenstock (1974) stated that increasing knowledge of cancer, which serves only to increase perceived benefits of prevention and early detection without simultaneously dealing with barriers to taking action, would have only marginal success. It is likely that such programmes would create conflict in many individuals who would find themselves highly motivated to both, take and avoid action.

The debate notwithstanding, most governments continue to develop programmes for screening and work on ways to improve screening rates, provided information is vital to any programme. Women require both information on the disease and information on the screening process itself (Jepson et al., 2007). Hence, researchers such as Sankarnarayan et al. (2007) have advocated education and engagement of the local communities as crucial factors in ensuring high participation. Baillie et al. (2004) suggested approaches that seek to work with the community and to connect cancer screening with a broader programme of community empowerment.

But research shows that providing general information about screening may not be helpful to all sections of the community especially for marginalized women (Nattinger et al., 1989; Champion, 1994; Skinner et al., 1994). Hence, variations in strategies need to be devised for women in different circumstances. For instance, community-based outreach programmes and integration of preventive services at the primary health care site, have been found to be effective for both African-American and Hispanic women. The use of mass media has been successful when targeted towards Hispanic women, but not towards African-American women. Elderly women respond well to mobile units and integration of preventive services at primary health care sites (Vellozzi et al., 1996). But the variations notwithstanding both screening and follow-up rates can be improved with interventions such as telephone and mail reminders from providers, multimedia educational interventions, peer counselling and financial incentives (Hewitt and Simone, 1999).

To improve the screening process, it is necessary to give primacy to various ethical principles. Screening policy makers now consider informed choice as important during screening programmes (as it prevents people from feeling coerced (National Screening Committee, 2000; Jepson et al., 2007)). Moreover, it is seen to have an economic advantage as it creates opportunities for selective screening based on individual risk profiles. Schwartz and Woloshin (2007) opined that women should be encouraged to decide what is right for them rather than being told what to do with regard to mammography screening.

Researchers have further suggested adhering to certain quality assurance principles during detection such as conducting cancer examination by a skilled, sympathetic doctor or nurse (RCOG, 2002) and incorporating the basic principles of respect, privacy, explanation and consent for intimate examinations (Coldicott et al., 2003).

Although these quality measures are easier to monitor in developed countries, in low-resource settings, screening programmes are hampered by poor infrastructure, absence of trained manpower, lack of quality control for laboratories and cytology reporting, poor treatment facilities and lack of education for women—all of which result in low participation. The Institute of Medicine (1999), recommends that low-resource countries that cannot afford the infrastructure required for organized screening programmes should focus on increasing awareness of signs and symptoms of cancer in the general population leading to early diagnosis and treatment.

In a developing country such as India, screening represents a greater challenge than it has been in more developed countries due to competing priorities and economic conditions. Sankarnarayan et al. (2007) showed the difficulty of achieving adequate coverage in screening programmes. Hence, they argued that the screening culture in the developed world may not be applicable in a developing country such as India. They have suggested affordable techniques for cancer screening such as clinical breast examination (CBE) and visual inspection with acetic acid (VIA) for cervical screening (Mittra, 1992; Sankarnarayan et al., 2007).

Okonkwo et al. (2008) found that the estimated cost-effectiveness of CBE screening for breast cancer in India compares favourably with that of mammography in developed countries and that the estimated mortality reduction was the greatest for programmes targeting women between the age of 40 and 60 years. Using a 3 per cent discount rate, a single CBE at age 50 years had an estimated cost-effectiveness ratio of Int.$793 per life year gained and a breast cancer mortality reduction of 2 per cent.

ACCESS AND BARRIERS TO SCREENING

Researchers have used the access and barrier perspectives to understand problems in the delivery of cancer care in various social settings. There are barriers to entry to care, which include characteristics of individuals and their social environment (such as poverty and socio-economic status, ethnic and racial characteristics and culture), and also characteristics of health care organization and financing (such as insurance coverage, regular source of care and service availability). Barriers within systems of care or treatment episodes include concerns about the ability to obtain needed and appropriate care, whether specialty care is available and whether care is provided appropriately, for example, according to recognized treatment guidelines and standards of care (Kasper, 2000).

The two most widely used models of access and barriers to care—the Behavioural Model of Health Services Use (Andersen, 1968; 1995; Aday and Andersen, 1975) and the Health Belief Model (Rosenstock, 1996; Strecher and Rosenstock, 1997)—have thrown light on the use of health care services including preventive health services and screening behaviour. It is generally assumed that if certain behavioural and structural changes are made, then people would automatically seek health care. But cultural issues and lay beliefs of people, influence patient's health-seeking behaviour—an area that has not received attention in cancer care management. Attention to cultural and psychosocial factors, such as health beliefs and attitudes that derive in part from culture, remains an underrepresented area in the literature on access and barriers to care (Albrecht et al., 2000).

Often, intricate personal processes of assessment and negotiation take place before someone decides to consult the doctor (Calnan, 1987). During this interim period, people draw upon lay ideas about health and illness from family and friends, media, current reading and so on.

With respect to cancer detection, studies have shown that lay ideas can delay cancer detection. For example, several researchers (Worden and Weisman, 1975; Adam et al., 1980; Mor et al., 1990; Ajekigbe, 1991) have reported that women did not realize the significance of a breast cancer symptom and often attributed it to a benign process. Moreover, erroneous beliefs about cancer can act as a barrier to access to early cancer detection or treatment services (Vernon et al., 1990; Jepson et al., 1991; Fajardo et al., 1992; Douglass et al., 1995). McKie (1995) in a study of English working-class women found that Pap smear was associated with sexual promiscuity, and hence women were reluctant to undergo it.

Besides lay beliefs, cultural norms also influence people undergoing screening. It is seen that participation in cancer screening conflicts with a strongly held cultural norm of female modesty as observed in the study of women of Mexican descent residing in Texas, USA (Borrayo and Jenkins, 2001). Similarly, Marks et al. (2008) showed that women are more likely to undergo cancer screening if they see a female rather than a male physician.

Cancer screening is also affected by socio-economic factors. Low level of education (which usually occurs in conjunction with low household income) is associated with lower cancer screening and re-screening (Rutledge et al., 1988; Mickey et al., 1997; Lannin et al., 1998). Researchers have shown that the use of cancer screening programmes is lower among women from low socio-economic backgrounds (Frazier et al., 1996). These women either lack knowledge on cancer screening or are less concerned about their health. Further, lack of knowledge, poor public health education and inadequate health care lead to poor access to cervical screening (Markovic et al., 2005). Many individuals know little about cancer and do not know that it can be successfully treated or why and when screening tests are useful (Myers et al., 1991; Grady et al., 1992). In studies of screening behaviour among Western women, higher education and income were important predictors of compliance (Centres for Disease Control, 1992; Champion and Miller, 1996). Aro et al. (1999) mentioned that individual-level determinants, such as social background, poor public health education, perceived risk and health behaviour, in general, can discourage people from going for screening.

Psychological factors may also impact screening rates. A study of Spanish women found that those with high fear of illness were less likely to participate in a cancer screening programme (Lostao et al., 2001). Researchers (Marks et al., 2008) indicated that the most frequently given reason for non-participation in cancer screening is that women do not feel it necessary as they were healthy.

Structural and organizational factors act as barriers in screening. For instance, many health systems and preventive programmes do not emphasize on early detection of cervical cancer (Ojanuga and Gilbert, 1992). It is observed that early detection of cancer is directly related to the access, quality and utilization of primary health care. For example, a study by Remennick (1999) showed that sparse contact between the immigrants and doctors resulted in the delayed detection of cancer. Moreover, absence of health facilities within a reasonable distance may make the screening tests inaccessible. Perhaps for this reason, residents of rural areas use cancer screening tests less often than their urban counterparts (Hayward et al., 1988; Katz and Hofer, 1994).

Further, structural barriers such as the absence of a regular source of care lead to lower rates of cancer screening (Zapka et al., 1992; Fox et al., 1994; Zapka, 1994; Bindman et al., 1996; Gordon et al., 1998). In a study of multiethnic black and Hispanic women in New York, breast and cervical cancer screening rates increased when women had a usual source of care and when they had a regular clinician at their usual source (O'Malley et al., 1997). However, among women with a regular source of care, Bindman et al. (1996) noted that several features of optimal primary care, including availability of care, continuity and communication, influenced significantly the receipt of breast and cervical cancer screening. These factors were independent of insurance status and patient socio-demographics.

ACCESS AND BARRIERS TO SCREENING IN ODISHA

Sociological studies on access and barriers to cancer screening are rare in India. This chapter presents the findings of a study on cancer management in Odisha (Pradhan, 2010) and provides information on the structural and organizational features of cancer awareness and screening programmes. The findings are based on field observation and interviews geared towards retrospective understanding of the problems faced by women patients, mostly from rural areas. These women, who belonged to low- and middle-income groups, were undergoing treatment at a Government Regional Cancer Hospital, namely Acharya Harihar Regional Cancer Centre (AHRCC). Secondary data consisted of annual reports and information, education and communication (IEC) materials of AHRCC.

CANCER CARE AT AHRCC: AWARENESS AND SCREENING

The AHRCC is one of the 25 Regional Cancer Centres (RCCs) in the country. In the year 1981, the erstwhile cancer wing of the SCB Medical College, Cuttack, was elevated to the level of RCC for conducting research, prevention of cancer and early detection and treatment. In 1984, this RCC became an autonomous institution, registered under the Societies Registration Act, 1860, and was named the AHRCC after the great Acharya Harihar, a dedicated social worker. AHRCC provides some of the components of cancer care beginning with primary prevention (awareness programmes), secondary prevention (screening and detection), diagnosis, treatment and end-of-life care.

Cancer detection in the state is primarily done through the District Cancer Control Programme (DCCP), which is one of the components of India's revised National Cancer Control Programme. AHRCC is the nodal agency for DCCP in the state and responsible for awareness and detection camps organized in the districts.

The site of the camp is decided by the Chief District Medical Officer (CDMO) or any non-governmental organization (NGO) participating in the programme. Although the camps organized under DCCP are usually conducted in a hospital, NGOs conduct these in schools or community halls. One closed room is selected for undertaking the screening of women-related cancers. In these camps, the doctors from AHRCC are invited based on their availability. Usually four to five doctors (including a lady doctor), two laboratory technicians, one pathologist and one sanitation worker are present in the camps. Technical support for the camp, including testing kits, is supplied by AHRCC.

Cancer-detection camps are also organized in districts, which are not under the direct control of DCCP by local NGOs. However, AHRCC's assistance is limited to providing technical expertise and supply of IEC material only. Financial provision is made by the NGOs from various health projects of Government of India or from voluntary contributions. AHRCC seems to be having little control and coordination with the NGOs, most of whom work autonomously and sporadically.

The doctors of AHRCC are not involved in the detection programmes on a regular basis. They participate in the detection camps only when invited by the CDMO of a particular district or by NGOs who have obtained funds from different Government health schemes. In the year 2005, merely three camps were organized; whereas in the year 2006, 10 camps were organized involving the doctors of AHRCC (Annual Report AHRCC, 2005–06).

Field observation shows that the holding of the screening camps is announced to the people of the locality by the health workers, the youth clubs or the NGO concerned two weeks prior to the organization of camps through leaflets, display of posters in the local hospital and by microphone announcements. After the initial announcement, the concerned medical staff/NGO registers the names of people who are interested in attending the camps. A pre-screening strategy is adopted to register only the names of those who complain of some cancer-related symptoms.

As far as the schedule of the camp is concerned, the first half of the camp is devoted to screening and detection. Clinical tests are conducted during the camps and reports delivered on the same day. Fine needle aspiration cytology (FNAC) and Pap smear tests are used for breast and cervial cancer screenings, respectively. The kits used for FNAC are syringe, needle, slides and ethyl alcohol (for fixative so that the cell architecture is not destroyed). The kits used for Pap smear are three to four speculums, brush for getting the smear from cervical canal, gloves, slides and ethyl alcohol. During the camps, women in the age group of 35–55 years are advised to have a Pap smear for cervical cancer at least once and seek further referral if any abnormality is detected. In case of breast cancer, the doctors advise breast self-examination (BSE) once every month with the help of demonstration made on leaflets and suggest consultation with gynaecologists if any symptom is noticed.

The second half of the day is devoted to awareness on cancer, wherein lectures are given with the help of audio-visual aids on major types of cancer, their symptoms, risk factors and prevention. The camps provide education and counselling related to lifestyle behaviours including smoking, tobacco, alcohol use, etc., and specific causes and symptoms of breast and cervical cancer. However, the duration of the camps is short, and there is no opportunity for clarification of doubts as lecture method is followed while explaining various types of cancer. During these camps, leaflets are also distributed among the participants. These leaflets, which are in the local language, contain information about symptoms of cancer and information for contacting the nearest health worker.

WHAT SEEMS TO BE GOING WRONG? CRITICAL REFLECTIONS

As is evident from the discussion above, camps seem to be conducted without much thought and preplanning, often in a rush to disburse the funds that anyway reach late to the organizers—be it the NGO or the AHRCC. As a result, they are inadequate, short in duration and organized without any systematic mapping and identification of the target group. Further, they do not cater to a defined population, selected according to age, gender and specific type of cancer.

As far as coverage is concerned, there seems to be no systematic mapping. This is clear from the fact that only three districts out of 30 in Odisha were covered under the DCCP at the time of study—the programme has been operational in the district of Balasore (since 1991–92) and in the districts of Jagatsinghpur and Khurda (since 1997–98).

As discussed earlier, adequate information and awareness are necessary for ensuring good screening participation rate. However, this is not the case as the study reveals. Apart from the DCCP, which anyway covered only three districts at the time of study, there was no other government programme to raise awareness and improve motivation for screening participation. Education related to lifestyle behaviours or counselling about risk factors for cancer occurrence was also not given. Besides, the use of mass media in awareness was conspicuous by its absence.

The mode of information was primarily textual and was not oriented to the needs of women who had poor educational level. But, these did not serve the needs of the better educated women either, since no elaboration was provided on the medical terminologies used. For instance, a brochure published by the ministry reads under signs and symptoms of cancer 'unusual bleeding or secretion' without clarifying what 'unusual' means.

Information leaflets were distributed arbitrarily, and although posters were displayed on the district hospitals, only those women who visited the hospital chanced to view them. Thirty per cent of the women in the sample (who belong to DCCP covered districts) had not even heard of them.

Information was also provided through oral mode, with microphones hosted on three wheelers. But this was largely localized and was not apparently a successful method of information dissemination.

The content of information was also not geared to the needs of the people. IEC components did not cater to the socially and economically disadvantaged, and rural–urban differences or differential needs of literate and illiterate women were overlooked.

Data reveal that out of a sample of 50 women cancer patients undergoing treatment at AHRCC, only 6 (12 per cent) were partially aware about cancer or its symptoms prior to their arrival at AHRCC. None of the 26 breast cancer patients had done BSE. Neither had they undergone clinical check-up for early detection of breast cancer. Similarly, among the 24 cervical cancer patients, none were aware about Pap smear test, before being detected with cervical cancer.

These data are in stark contrast to the government's policy of reducing occurrence of cancer through health education, early detection and diagnosis by screening methods and self-examination. None of the women were aware about screening programmes in their locality. Even women staying in urban settings where DCCP is operational were not aware about screening camps for cancer detection.

Although 22 per cent of the sample had passed school education, their awareness of risk factors and screening techniques was equally poor and they did not have any comparable advantage over the uneducated women. Further, no variation in response of the respondents was noted according to demographic factors such as location, age, marital status, employment and economic status.

Therefore, it seems that poor awareness of cancer has acted as a barrier in the screening and early detection of cancer. Hence, in response to the question 'Have you attended any screening programme before coming to AHRCC?', none of the women gave reply in the affirmative.

A woman of 50 years staying in a village in Balasore District, which comes under the DCCP, remarked rather sarcastically:

> Prior to having this disease, nobody in our locality even knew about cancer. So why go for screening camps? We are staying in a town of Balasore District but still we do not know that after a certain age women should do Pap test for screening of cervical cancer. The ASHA didi (community health worker) who discusses with us about our health problems has also not discussed with us about this .... (Stage Ib, Cervical Cancer)

In response to the question 'Would you have gone for screening if you were aware of cancer and if facilities were available in your locality?', 94 per cent of respondents answered in the affirmative. When these women were further asked 'What factors in your opinion would motivate women to attend screening programmes?', they cited a few enabling factors mentioned in Table 4.1.

Table 4.1 shows that the majority (92 per cent) of the respondents required prior information about cancer and its symptoms in local language, followed by awareness on the importance of screening and screening process (88 per cent). Women believed that such information help them recognize the symptoms and understand the gravity of the disease and the need for medical consultation. They also

Table 4.1 Womens' Reporting of Enabling Factors for Screening Participation

Enabling Factors	*Number of Respondents N = 50*
Prior information about cancer and its symptoms in local language	46 (92%)
Awareness on importance of screening for early diagnosis of cancer and the screening process itself	44 (88%)
Adequate facilities for screening near to their home	40 (80%)
Delivery of test reports on the same day	40 (80%)

expressed the need for screening to be located near to their homes (80 per cent), and test reports to be delivered on the same day of screening (80 per cent). The presence of female doctors was another enabling factor (76 per cent) cited by the respondents. Finally, 40 per cent women were of the opinion that incentives in terms of certain monetary benefits would have motivated them for screening.

Coming back to the structural and organizational features, frequency of camps was another feature not handled adequately. The camps appeared to be a just one-time affair of short duration (from 9 am to 4 pm). They were organized once in each area with no special effort being made to include population excluded from these camps, or through contact-tracing to help women undergo repeat tests at recommended intervals.

Perhaps, the most glaring lacunae lay in the fact that the camps were not gender specific—both men and women were enrolled—but discussion on women-related cancers was restricted to half an hour only. Hence, it is doubtful as to how far women with low educational levels could actually understand the symptoms of cancer and take remedial measures. Moreover, these camps were not interactive and did not provide an adequate forum to clarify doubts. It is not surprising that many women felt discouraged, particularly when they had to travel from far-off places to attend the camps.

Compounding these problems is the fact that ethical principles such as informed consent and anonymity were hardly adhered to during these camps.

Follow-up measures after screening camps were equally poor. These were not equipped to help women seek immediate consultation with local-level practitioners because of poor available expertise.

Those identified with clinical problems were advised to seek help at AHRCC for further diagnosis and treatment, but there were no strategies—financial and logistical—to enable them to do so. This raises serious ethical questions about the necessity of organizing the camps in the absence of adequate follow-up procedures. These questions attain greater significance given the serious socio-cultural barriers faced by the women.

SOCIO-CULTURAL BARRIERS

The study shows that preventive behaviour, in general, was highly influenced by the social positioning of women in the society. Majority (78 per cent) of the patients admitted to AHRCC were from rural pockets of Odisha with 48 per cent belonging to families below the poverty line.

A large number of these patients (64 per cent) were in the reproductive age group (18–50 years) with 94 per cent of them being married. But they were unable to take independent decisions perhaps due to poor education (62 per cent respondents were below matriculate and 16 per cent of the respondents were uneducated), economic dependence (only 20 per cent were working women) and cultural norms.

Seventy-two per cent depended on male members in going for health check-up; 28 per cent gave priority to household responsibilities over their own health. Fifty-six per cent respondents belonged to nuclear families with little support in the care-giving process and multiple roles in the family left them with little time for their own health care. Moreover, these women had grown up believing in their identity as caregivers and had difficulty in enlisting the help of male members for their own health concerns.

Lay beliefs also influenced preventive behaviour. As already observed, very few women were aware about the symptoms of breast or cervical cancer. Hence, despite noticing some bodily changes, they did not seek medical advice. Majority (80.77 per cent) had observed a small eruption or lump in the breast, whereas others felt a swelling of breast (11.54 per cent) or were unable to lift the arm (7.69 per cent). Similarly, in case of cervical cancer, majority (75 per cent) had observed abnormal bleeding or white discharge, whereas others noticed blood in stool (16.67 per cent) or felt pain in the lower abdomen and hardening of the stomach (8.33 per cent). Thus, despite identifying these bodily disturbances, they did not attribute the symptoms to any 'disease'.

One of the reasons for their failure to attribute pathology to bodily changes was lay notions of illness, which differed greatly from biomedical etiologies of cancer. Women's responses were embedded in local life perspectives on illness and cultural assumptions of disease and dignified approach/response to it. For instance, two women (7.69 per cent) with swelling of the breasts thought it could be due to pregnancy. Some women (23.07 per cent) felt too shy to discuss problems about their private parts, and hence kept the initial symptoms of the disease to themselves. Women having heavy bleeding misconstrued it as menopause (16.66 per cent), whereas others (20.83 per cent) felt that it 'just happens with many women'. Similarly, 8.33 per cent of them mentioned 'such things are not disclosed to others'. One woman who had blood in stool attributed it to summer 'heat' while another women attributed abdominal pain to gastritis complications. Almost 27 per cent undermined the significance of the symptoms and deffered consulting a doctor for health check-up. Some felt that there was no need for medical check-up in the absence of pain (27.56 per cent). Some of the ways in which women understood and expressed the initial symptoms of cancer are presented further.

One 70-year-old woman came from Balasore District who was detected with cervical cancer narrated:

> I had drops of blood coming whenever I passed stool. I thought it might be due to the fact that it was summer and my stomach has got heated up ... Without disclosing my problem to anyone, I drank lots of water and splashed it on my stomach too. But when it continued for one month, I could not hide my fear and anxiety and told my daughter-in-law who took me to a lady doctor in Cuttack for check-up. (Stage III, Cervix Cancer)

Another woman from Bolangir District aged 50 years misjudged the symptoms of bleeding:

> One year back my stomach felt big and I began to gain weight. There was pain in the abdomen and bleeding in-between periods. I was in the late 40s and I had heard that at menopause such bleeding takes place among women. So I kept the information to myself. The thought of having cancer never occurred to me. I did not know anything about it and neither was aware about any screening camps being organized in our locality. (Stage IIa, Cervix Cancer)

These narratives show that despite noticing bodily changes, women drew upon local health beliefs to explain their ailments.

One married woman, aged 55 years from Nayagarh District (about 90 km from Cuttack), noticed a lump in her left breast. She described her condition thus:

> There was a lump in left breast which used to move when pressed, it was a solid mass. At that time our house was under construction in our village. I was busy in doing household work and providing food to the labourers who were working. I asked the Anganwadi didi who organizes meetings of our SHG. She said it must be a swelling due to the heat. I also did not disclose this to my husband as there was no pain. (Stage IIIa, Breast Cancer)

When enquired whether she knew that a small lump could lead to breast cancer, she replied:

> Women are busy with so many household activities. Where is the time to think about one's own health? Besides, as women we need someone to take us to the doctor. I thought, for such a small problem, why should I request my husband to take me to the hospital nearly 5 kilometres away from our home?

The persistence of lay beliefs in the sample betray poor outcome of the awareness programmes run by the government. They also indicate the urgency to address these beliefs through sensitive design of health communication messages.

ETHICS OF CANCER DETECTION IN RESOURCE-POOR SETTINGS: A BOON OR A BANE?

The findings of the study raise serious doubts about the efficacy of screening programmes in Odisha. Findings show structural and organizational, as well as socio-cultural barriers that prevent the emergence of a sound prevention strategy for cancer. Given the fact that in a poor state such as Odisha, mass screening programmes at regular intervals are financially not feasible, a proper systematization becomes important in terms of coverage, frequency, age and gender specificity. Moreover, serious thought has to be given to the selection of a proper screening test that is cost effective and efficacious and that provides a realistic match between available resources and their universal and uniform availability for the population. It may be mentioned here that it is now well recognized that conventional exfoliative cervicovaginal cytology, that is, Pap smear has serious limitations in Indian setting and viable alternatives need to be explored (see Kerkar and Kulkarni, 2006; in Takiar, 2010). Similarly, the challenge involved in CBE screening in India, and how it compares with mamography in developed countries in terms of mortality reduction and cost effectiveness, need serious thinking (see Moss, 2008). Currently, even data on reduction of mortality by mammographic screening remain ambivalent (Callies and Oberhoff, 2005).

Lacking more scientific inputs on screening techniques, there is a risk of causing psychological harm to the population—a point raised by researchers in Western countries (Rimer and Bluman, 1997; Aro et al., 2000; Irwig et al., 2006; Jepson et al., 2007). Moreover, lack of adherence to strict international quality assurance guidelines, both clinical and ethical, creates serious complexities as far as the very desirability of screening programmes are concerned.

These limitations notwithstanding, if one continues to repose faith on screening as a method of reducing cancer mortality in India, we need to critically examine the socio-cultural determinants with the intent of using them as a 'resource' rather than as a 'barrier'. This is especially true for awareness programmes for improving screening participation rates. These need more serious design by incorporating IEC contents in local dialect and suited to population characteristics.

As noted by scholars in the West, more sensitive participatory methods have to be evolved (Irwig et al., 2006; Jepson et al., 2007). Taking the assistance of women groups for cancer screening as suggested by Milic (2004) and creating supportive social networks may positively influence cancer screening practices among women (Suarez et al., 1994; Howson, 1999; Kelsey et al., 2000). An important suggestion in this regard is to connect the cancer-detection programme with broader programmes of empowerment of women through self-help groups (SHGs) in the villages and by taking the services of the ASHA and *Anganwadi* workers. Structurally, this means integration of cancer-detection programmes with the existing health structure in Odisha starting from the sub-health centre, primary health centre and community health centre at the village level to the district and state levels. In other words, training in oncology is necessary at different hierarchical levels.

One may mention here that a hierarchical structure of health delivery already exists in Odisha. Yet, AHRCC has made little attempt to take organizational advantage of these groups and the existing structure for its mandate on awareness and detection of cancer. It has also been unable to integrate cancer control programmes with other health programmes in the state such as NRHM or develop specific collaborations with the existing women-oriented programmes. For instance, the Mission Shakti programme of the Government of Odisha promotes women SHGs in each village with the help of Anganwadi workers. Each SHG has around 15–20 women within its group. At present, there are 367,029 SHGs in 30 districts of Odisha with a total membership of 44 lakh women (Mission Shakti Brochure, 2009) who could be adequately trained in primary and secondary prevention activities.

However, the ethical complexities do not end here. Eventually, one has to pose a more serious question: What is the approach to the management of an abnormal screening? In resource-poor places such as Odisha, does the state have adequate provision for proper diagnosis and treatment? In other words, if continuity of care in terms of definitive diagnosis and treatment cannot be ensured, the entire effort in primary and secondary prevention activities is rendered futile. Assessing the level of structural competence in ensuring a good follow-up procedure would be an honest approach to judicious management of meagre resources.

REFERENCES

Adam, S.A., J.K. Homer and M.P. Vessev, 1980, 'Delay in Treatment for Breast Cancer', *Community Medicine*, 2: i95.

Aday, L. and R.M. Andersen, 1975, *Development of Indices of Access to Medical Care*. Ann Arbour, MI: Health Administration Press.

Ajekigbe, A.T., 1991, 'Fear of Mastectomy: The Most Common Factor Responsible for Late Presentation of Carcinoma of the Breast in Nigeria', *Clinical Oncology*, 3: 78.

Albrecht, G.L., R. Fitzpatrick and S.C. Scrimshaw (Eds.), 2000, *Handbook of Social Studies in Health and Medicine*. London: Sage Publication.

Andersen, R.M., 1968, *Behavioural Model of Families Use of Health Services*. Research Series No.25, Chicago, IL: Centre for Health Administration Studies, University of Chicago.

Andersen, R.M., 1995, 'Revisiting the Behavioral Model and Access to Medical Care: Does it Matter?' *Journal of Health and Social Behavior*, 36: 1–10.

Aro, A.R., P.S. Absetz, T.M. van Elderen, E. van der Ploeg and L.J.T. van der Kamp, 2000, 'False-Positive Findings in Mammography Screening Induce Short-Term Distress – Breast Cancer – Specific Concern Prevails Longer', *European Journal of Cancer*, 36: 1089–97.

Aro, A.R., H.J. de Koning, P. Absetz and M. Schreck, 1999, 'Psychosocial Predictors of First Attendance for Organized Mammography Screening', *Journal of Medical Screening*, 6: 82–8.

Baillie, L., S. Broughton, J. Bassett-Smith, W. Aasen, M. Oostinde, B.A. Marino and K. Hewitt, 2004, 'Community Health, Community Involvement, and Community Empowerment: Too Much to Expect?', *Journal of Community Psychology*, 32: 217–28.

Bindman, A.B., K. Grumbach, D. Osmond, K. Vranizan and A.L. Stewart, 1996, 'Primary Care Receipt of Preventive Services', *Journal of General Internal Medicine*, 11(5): 269–76.

Borrayo, E.A. and S.R. Jenkins, 2001, 'Feeling Indecent: Breast Cancer Screening Resistance of Mexican-Descent Women', *Journal of Health Psychology*, 6: 49–57.

Callies, R. and C. Oberhoff, 2005, 'Pros and Cons of Early Cancer Detection in Breast Carcinoma', *MMW Fortschritte der Medizin*, 147(14): 30–2.

Calnan, M., 1987, *Health and Illness: The Lay Perspective*. London: Tavistock.

Centres for Disease Control, 1992, 'Cancer Screening Behaviour among US Women: Breast Cancer, 1987–89', *Morbidity and Mortality Weekly Review*, 41: 26–7.

Champion, V.L., 1994, 'Strategies to Increase Mammography Utilization', *Medical Care*, 32(2): 118–29.

Champion, V.L. and A.M. Miller, 1996, 'Recent Mammography in Women Aged 35 and Older: Predisposing Variables', *Health Care for Women International*, 17: 233–45.

Clasen, C.M., S.W. Vernon, P.D. Mullen and G.L. Jackson, 1994, 'A Survey of Physician Beliefs and Self-Reported Practices Concerning Screening for Early Detection of Cancer', *Social Science & Medicine*, 39(6): 841–49.

Coldicott, Y., C. Pope and C. Roberts, 2003, 'The Ethics of Intimate Examinations-Teaching Tomorrow's Doctors', *British Medical Journal*, 326: 97–101.

Douglass, M., A. Bartolucci, J. Waterbor and A. Sirles, 1995, 'Breast Cancer Early Detection: Differences Between African American and White Women's Health Beliefs and Detection Practices', *Oncology Nursing Forum*, 22: 835–37.

Fajardo, L.L., M. Saint-Germain, T.J. Meakem, C. Rose and B.J. Hillman, 1992, 'Factors Influencing Women to Undergo Screening Mammography', *Radiology*, 184: 59–63.

Fletcher, S.W., W. Black, H. Harris, B.K. Rimer and S. Shapiro, 1993, 'Report of the International Workshop on Screening for Breast Cancer', *Journal of National Cancer Institute*, 85: 1644–56.

Fox, S.A., A.L. Siu and J.A. Stein, 1994, 'The Importance of Physician Communication on Breast Cancer Screening of Older Women', *Archives of Internal Medicine*, 154: 2058–68.

Frazier, E.L., R.B. Jiles and R. Mayberry, 1996, 'Use of Screening Mammography and Clinical Breast Examination among Black, Hispanic and White Women', *Preventive Medicine*, 25: 118–25.

Gordon, N.P., T.G. Rundall and L. Parker, 1998, 'Type of Health Care Coverage and the Likelihood of Being Screened for Cancer', *Medical Care*, 36(5): 636–45.

Grady, K.E., J.P. Lemkau, J.M. McVay and S.T. Reisine, 1992, 'The Importance of Physician Encouragement in Breast Cancer Screening of Older Women', *Preventive Medicine*, 21: 766–80.

Hayward, R.A., M.F. Shapiro, H.E. Freeman and C.R. Corey, 1988, 'Who Gets Screened for Cervical and Breast Cancer?', *Archives of Internal Medicine*, 148: 1177–81.

Hewitt, M. and J. Simone (Eds.), 1999, 'The Institute of Medicine Report. Access to Cancer Care'. In *Ensuring Quality Cancer Care*, Washington, DC: National Academy Press, p. 55.

Howson, A., 1999, 'Cervical Screening, Compliance and Moral Obligation', *Sociology of Health and Illness*, 21(4): 401–25.

Institute of Medicine Report, 1999, In *Ensuring Quality Cancer Care*, edited by M. Hewitt and J. Simone, Washington, DC: National Academy Press.

Irwig, L., K. McCaffery, G. Salkeld and P. Bossuyt, 2006, 'Informed Choice for Screening: Implications for Evaluation', *British Medical Journal*, 332: 1148–50.

Jepson, C., L.G. Kessler, B. Portnoy and T. Gibbs, 1991, 'Black-White Differences in Cancer Prevention Knowledge and Behaviour', *American Journal of Public Health*, 81: 501–04.

Jepson, R.G., J. Hewison, A. Thompson and D. Weller, 2007, 'Patient Perspectives on Information and Choice in Cancer Screening: A Qualitative Study in the UK', *Social Science & Medicine*, 65: 890–99.

Kasper, J.D., 2000, 'Health-Care Utilization and Barriers to Health Care'. In *Handbook of Social Studies in Health and Medicine*, edited by G.L. Albrecht, R. Fitzpatrick and S.C. Scrimshaw, London: Sage Publication.

Katz, S.J. and T.P. Hofer, 1994, 'Socioeconomic Disparities in Preventive Care Persist Despite Universal Coverage. Breast and Cervical Cancer Screening in Ontario and the United States', *Journal of the American Medical Association*, 272(7): 530–34.

Kelsey, J.L. and L. Bernstein, 1996, 'Epidemiology and Prevention of Breast Cancer', *Annual Review of Public Health*, 17: 47–67.

Kelsey, K.S., M.K. Campbell, I. Tessaro, S. Benedict, L. Belton, L.M. Fernandez, C. Henriquez-Roldan and B. DeVellis, 2000, 'Social Support and Health Behaviours among Blue-Collar Women Workers', *American Journal of Health Behaviour*, 24(6): 434–43.

Kerkar, R.A. and Y.V. Kulkarni, 2006, 'Screening for Cervical Cancer: An Overview', *Journal of Obstetrics and Gynecology India*, 56(2): 115–22.

Lannin, D.R., H.F. Mathews and J. Mitchell, 1998, 'Influence of Socioeconomic and Cultural Factors on Racial Differences in Late-Stage Presentation of Breast Cancer', *Journal of the American Medical Association*, 279: 1801–07.

Lostao, L., T.E. Joner, J.W. Pettit, P. Chorot and B. Sandin, 2001, 'Health Beliefs and Illness Attitudes as Predictors of Breast Cancer Screening Attendance', *European Journal of Public Health*, 11: 274–79.

Mandelblatt, J., H. Freeman and D. Winczewski, 1997, 'The Costs and Effects of Cervical Cancer Screening in a Public Hospital Emergency Room', *American Journal of Public Health*, 87(7): 1182–89.

Markovic, M., V. Kesic, L. Topic and B. Matejic, 2005, 'Barriers to Cervical Screening: A Qualitative Study with Women in Serbia', *Social Science & Medicine*, 61: 2528–35.

Marks, D.V., M. Murray, B. Evans, C. Willig, C. Woodall and C.M. Sykes, 2008, *Immunization and Screening in Health Psychology: Theory Research and Practice*, 2nd ed. New Delhi: Sage.

McKie, L., 1995, 'The Art of Surveillance or Reasonable Prevention? The Case of Cervical Screening', *Sociology of Health and Illness*, 17: 441–57.

Mickey, R.M., J.L. Vezina, J.K. Worden and S.L. Warner, 1997, 'Breast Screening Behaviour and Interactions with Health Care Providers among Lower Income Women', *Medical Care*, 35(12): 1204–11.

Milic, A., 2004, 'The Women's Movement in Serbia and Montenegro at the Turn of the Millennium: A Sociological Study of Women's Groups', *Feminist Review*, 76: 65–82.

Mission Shakti Brochure, 2009, *Pragati Pathe Mission Shakti. Brochure Distributed in a Meeting*. Government of Orissa.

Mittra, I., 1992, 'Screening for Breast Cancer', *World Health Forum*, 13(1): 277–85.

Mor, V., S. Masterson-Allen, R. Goldberg, E. Guadagnoli and M.S. Wool, 1990, 'Pre-Diagnostic Symptom Recognition and Help Seeking among Cancer Patients', *Journal of Community Health*, 15: 253.

Moss, Sue, 2008, 'Screening for Breast Cancer in India—Is It An Appropriate Strategy?', *Journal of National Cancer Institute*, 100(18): 1270–71.

Myers, R.E., E.A. Ross and T.A. Wolf, 1991, 'Behavioural Interventions to Increase Adherence in Colorectal Cancer Screening', *Medical Care*, 29: 1039–50.

National Screening Committee, 1998, *First Report of the UK National Screening Committee*. London: Department of Health.

National Screening Committee, 2000, *Second Report of the National Screening Committee*, [online] available at http://www.nsc.nhs.uk/library/lib_ind.htm.

Nattinger, A.B., R.J. Panzer and J. Janus, 1989, 'Improving the Utilization of Screening Mammography in Primary Care Practices', *Archives of Internal Medicine*, 149: 2087–92.

O'Malley, A.S., J. Mandelblatt and K. Gold, 1997, 'Continuity of Care and the Use of Breast and Cervical Cancer Screening Services in a Multiethnic Community', *Archives of Internal Medicine*, 157(13): 1462–70.

Ojanuga, D.N. and C. Gilbert, 1992, 'Women's Access to Health Care in Developing Countries', *Social Science and Medicine*, 35(4): 613–17.

Okonkwo, Q.L., G. Draisma, A. der Kinderen, M.L. Brown and H.J. de Koning, 2008, 'Breast Cancer Screening Policies in Developing Countries: A Cost-Effectiveness Analysis for India', *Journal of National Cancer Institute*, 100(18): 1290–300.

Pradhan, S., 2010, 'Cancer Management at the Regional Cancer Centre in Orissa: Women's Experience of Breast and Cervix Cancer Care'. Thesis submitted to Indian Institute of Technology, Kharagpur for the award of the degree Doctor of Philosophy.

Remennick, L.I., 1999, 'Preventive Behaviour among Recent Immigrants: Russian Speaking Women and Cancer Screening in Israel', *Social Science & Medicine*, 48: 1669–84.

Rimer, B.K. and L.G. Bluman, 1997, 'The Psychosocial Consequences of Mammography', *Journal of the National Cancer Institute Monograph*, 22: 131–38.

Rosenstock, I.M., 1974, 'Historical Origins of the Health Belief Model'. In *The Health Belief Model and Personal Health Behaviour*, edited by M.H. Becker, Thorofare, NJ: Charles B. Slack, pp. 1–8.

Rosenstock, I.M., 1996, 'Why People Use Health Services', *Milbank Memorial Fund Quarterly*, 44: 94–124.

Royal College of Obstetricians and Gynaecologists (RCOG), 2002, *Gynaecological Examinations: Guidelines for Special Practice*. London: RCOG.

Rutledge, D.N., W.H. Hartmann, P.O. Kinman and A.C. Winfield, 1988, 'Exploration of Factors Affecting Mammography Behaviours', *Preventive Medicine*, 17: 412–22.

Sankarnarayan, R., P.O. Esmy and R. Rajkumar, 2007, 'Effect of Visual Screening on Cervical Cancer Incidence and Mortality in Tamil Nadu, India: A Cluster Randomized Trail', *The Lancet*, 370: 398–406.

Schwartz, L.M. and S. Woloshin, 2007, 'Participation in Mammography Screening', *British Medical Journal*, 335: 731.

Shapiro, S., E.A. Coleman and M. Broeders, 1998, 'Breast Cancer Screening Programs in 22 Countries: Current Policies, Administration and Guidelines', *International Journal of Epidemiology*, 27: 735–42.

Skinner, C.S., V.J. Strecher and H. Hospers, 1994, 'Physician's Recommendations for Mammography: Do Tailored Messages Make a Difference?', *American Journal of Public Health*, 84: 43–9.

Strecher, V.J. and I.M. Rosenstock, 1997, 'The Health Belief Model'. In *Health Behaviour and Health Education: Theory Research and Practice*, 2nd ed., edited by K. Glanz, F.M. Lewis and B.K. Rimer, San Francisco, CA: Jossey-Bass.

Strong, K., N. Wald, A. Miller and A. Alwan, 2005, 'WHO Consultation Group. Current Concepts in Screening for Non-Communicable Disease: World Health Organization Consultation Group Report on Methodology of Non-Communicable Disease Screening', *Journal of Medical Screening*, 12: 12–19.

Suarez, L., L. Lloyd, N. Weiss, T. Rainbolt and L. Pulley, 1994, 'Effect of Social Networks on Cancer-Screening Behaviour of Older Mexican-American Women', *Journal of National Cancer Institute*, 86(10): 775–79.

Takiar, R., D. Nadayil and A. Nandakuma, 2010, 'Projections of Number of Cancer Cases in India (2010-2020) by Cancer Groups Research Communication', *Asian Pacific Journal of Cancer Prevention*, 11: 1045–49.

Vellozzi, C.J., M. Romans and R.B. Rothenberg, 1996, 'Delivering Breast and Cervical Cancer Screening Services to Underserved Women: Part I. Literature Review and Telephone Survey', *Women's Health Issues*, 6(2): 65–73.

Vernon, S.W., E.A. Laville and G.L. Jackson, 1990, 'Participation in Breast Screening Programs: A Review', *Social Science & Medicine*, 30: 1107–18.

Wilson, J.M.C. and G. Jungner, 1968, *The Principles and Practice of Screening for Disease*. Geneva: WHO.

Worden, J.W. and A.D. Weisman, 1975, 'Psychosocial Components of Lagtime in Cancer Diagnosis', *Journal of Psychosomatic Research* 19: 69.

Zapka, J.G., 1994, 'Promoting Participation in Breast Cancer Screening', *American Journal of Public Health*, 84(1): 12–13.

Zapka, J.G., D. Hosmer and M.E. Costanza, 1992, 'Changes in Mammography Use: Economic, Need and Service Factors', *American Journal of Public Health*, 82: 1345–51.

CHAPTER 5

Contextualizing Maternal and Child Health in India: From Colonial Era to Globalized Era

Afzal Sayeed

Matri Devo Bhava[1]

Health and well-being of citizens is the most valuable asset for any country, and their care is the most sacred commitment of any government. The development of any society can be measured by the quality of health care delivery services in general and maternal and child health care in particular. Maternal and child health (MCH) are natural corollaries of each other, which refer to the health of women during pregnancy, childbirth, postpartum care, etc., and care of relatively more vulnerable newborns and children from malnutrition, infectious disease, etc. The broader view incorporates the social determinants of health that are considered critical for attaining high standards of MCH and development.

India, the largest democracy of the world, with great diversity and a population of 121 million, is an age-old civilization, but as a just over 60-year-old young independent nation came a long way in developing health care infrastructure and services. The colonial era was marked by more individual voluntary efforts that lacked organized planning pertaining to MCH. India, on attaining independence, embarked upon the 'socialist pattern' of planned development and the health services, as 'the foundation of all things' found key attention for the socio-economic development process.

The social policy is considered a reflection of the nation's concern for the welfare of its citizens. The changes in policy over time that a state follows in order to improve the outcomes are inevitable. We came a long way in terms of the number of years of providing services but not significantly in the form of bringing qualitative improvement in the health service delivery process and MCH services are no exception. This chapter is an attempt to go into the annals of historical development in the realm of MCH situations, policy, programme and outcomes.

HEALTH SERVICES FOR MOTHERS AND CHILDREN DURING COLONIAL PERIOD

Nearly one-half of the total deaths at all ages in British India had taken place among children under 10 years of age; of these, nearly half of the deaths were among infants under one year (Table 5.1). A conservative estimate of the annual number of deaths among women in the reproductive ages from causes associated with pregnancy and childbearing is 200,000; whereas the number of women who had to undergo, every year, varying degrees of disability and suffering from the same causes is about four million if the ratio of morbidity to mortality considered reasonable elsewhere can be applied to India (Bhore, 1946).

According to National Planning Committee Report (1948) 'The health of the people depends primarily upon the social and environmental conditions under which they live and work, upon security against fear and want, upon nutritional standards, upon educational facilities, and the facilities for exercise and leisure.'

Initially, during the colonial period, the policies confined to the question of essential services to protect the health of mother and children. These services were expected to provide little antenatal supervision; skilled assistance at childbirth, including institutional facilities where necessary; and meagre health protection to children from birth through the successive stages of infancy, early and late childhood.

The growth of maternity and child welfare work has been mainly because of voluntary efforts due to the lack of an organized programme of development in this domain.

Table 5.1 Infant Mortality Rate during British India

	Year	*Sex*	*0–1 year*	*15–40 years*
British India	1930–32	Male	184.4	31.0
		Female	167.1	35.8

DEVELOPMENT OF MATERNITY AND CHILD WELFARE IN INDIA

Studies on health services in British India reveal that the evolution of general health services was the outcome of the interests of the British army and later the political interests of the colonial government (Jeffrey, 1988). A popular notion is that the wives who came to India along with Viceroys and officers got involved in social work not on a professional basis, rather purely on a humanitarian basis and provided their services in British India. Even at the end of the nineteenth century, one-third of the 343 women doctors with British degrees in British India were from overseas (Shah, 1948).

The motion started with attempts made by the Women Missionaries from Britain to train the indigenous *Dais* for the practice of better standards of midwifery than those existing accustomed practice. The earliest attempt in this direction was made by Miss Hewlett of the Church of England Zenana Mission in 1866.

In 1885, the Dufferin Fund Committee was established with the objective of providing medical aid to the women of India through women doctors. The Dufferin Fund came into existence due to the interest and initiatives of a missionary doctor, Ms Bielby, who came to India in 1875 and opened a dispensary, and then a small hospital in Lucknow. In 1881, when Ms Bielby was going to England for her higher studies, the Maharaja of Poona (now called as Pune) requested her to visit her old patient the Maharani of Punna. During the visit, the Maharani gave her a gold chain with a locket. Inside the locket was a note stating the sufferings and complications faced by the Indian women at the time of childbirth. Ms Bielby was asked to deliver the chain personally to the Queen of England. On receiving the message, the Queen asked many questions and enquired about the conditions and sufferings of the Indian women. When Lady Dufferin came to India in 1883, the Queen ordered her to arrange for medical aid for the women of India. This paved way for the creation of the Dufferin fund (Qadeer, 2011).

The Dufferin fund along with a little financial support from the Government of India opened the Lady Reading Health School in 1918 at Delhi for the training of the health visitors for providing public health services, MCH services and to supervise auxiliary nurse midwives (ANMs).

Along with this initiative, the 'Medical Women for India' fund was initiated in 1882, which invited medical practitioners from abroad to come and work in India. The fund was created at the private initiative of Indian and American businessmen. Later, in the early twentieth century, Lady Curzon's Victoria Memorial Scholarship and Lady Reading Women of India Fund for running a maternity hospital in Shimla came up in 1903. In 1919, the Lady Chelmsford All-India League for maternity and child welfare was founded, which collected funds for mother and child welfare and established demonstration services on an all-India basis.

In 1930, under the aegis of Red Cross Society, a 'Maternal and Child Welfare Bureau' was established with the objective of promoting maternity and child welfare work throughout the country. The next milestone was the establishment of a training curriculum in the All India Institute of Hygiene and Public Health, Calcutta (Kolkata), in 1933, which qualifies women doctors for a diploma in maternity and child welfare.

Although maternity services provided through charity organizations under the aegis of qualified British women catered to the needs of the upper-middle-class women, majority of the women (depended) on the maligned traditional *Dai*. The number of deliveries performed by *Dais* was more in comparison to institutionalized deliveries. Later, these institutions started discrediting the traditional systems and practices of the *Dais* and portrayed them as being ignorant, vicious and careless, and thus they were able to establish the superiority of allopathic maternity practices. The colonial government instead of preserving the strength of traditional practices followed by *Dais*, introduced training programmes, based entirely on British curricula. Apart from discrediting the traditional *Dais*, the patrons of the Lady Dufferin Fund also blamed the '*purdah* system' as a retrogressive practice of an inferior culture for their poor health.

The colonial government thus encouraged the growth of institutionalized maternity care through British women professionals who were permitted to practise and run the hospitals and dispensaries. These institutionalized maternity services created an opportunity for Western women professionals, who were finding it difficult to get a break in male-dominated profession in their own countries as well as the means of entry into the medical schools, becoming eminent practitioners by showing their work experiences gained in India. However, their work was purely projected as philanthropic activity, and thus health remained as an external arena of the health policies of the colonial rule.

The Indian professionals who were active in the national movement with the support of the overseas professionals ultimately succeeded in exerting sufficient political pressure on the colonial government for playing proactive role in the health sector. Finally, in 1942, a National Committee was set up to examine health issues in India.

Personnel and Infrastructural Deficit

In 1943, according to the Bhore Committee Report, there were 5,000 practicing midwives in the country with an increment of only 300 qualified professionals annually. However, for a total of probably 10 million births each year in British India, nearly 100,000 midwives were required for making a huge gap on the basis of one midwife for every 100 births.

The total number of health visitors in the same period was 700–750. The qualification of these health workers ranges from third standard from Anglo-vernacular school to as high as matriculation differing from state to state. There were seven training centres located at Delhi, Lucknow, Calcutta (Kolkata), Madras (Chennai), Poona (Pune), Bombay (Mumbai) and Nagpur providing training for 6–18 months and generating 60 professionally qualified health visitors annually. The role of the health visitors was to supervise the work of five midwives, thus making a deficit of 17,500 health visitors to control the work of 100,000 midwives.

The total number of women doctors including graduates and licentiates was not supposed to exceed 4,000. Out of these, about a thousand were engaged in public sector, whereas another thousand were not practising due to some reason. The remaining were in general practice concentrated in the urban areas only, thus making rural vulnerable group of women and children doubly marginalized. The total number of women doctors with special training in this branch of health administration is only about a dozen medical graduates and about 50 or 60 licentiates.

Before independence, in most parts of the country, maternity and child welfare centres were run by health visitors. Madras and Delhi were the only provinces where women doctors were employed in both rural and urban areas. In 1942, Madras was the first province to initiate a programme to organize the existing maternity and child welfare work in a systematic manner. A total of 14 district boards and 32 municipalities maintained 225 centres, which employed 51 women medical officers, 32 health visitors and 422 midwives. A total of 7,900 clinics were held and 53,100 deliveries attended by qualified midwives and a total of about a million home visits were made. Even then, only about 3 per cent of the total births could be reached by the organization where the services had been best developed.

MATERNITY AND CHILD HEALTH PROGRAMMES AFTER INDEPENDENCE

With the end of colonial rule in India, the population of the country expected a radical transformation of the exploitative social structure that the British rule had nurtured and consolidated. But these expectations were belied as the new rulers were mere indigenous substitute for the colonial masters.

According to Indian Constitution, only civil and political rights are justifiable, whereas social and economic rights such as health are under the Directive Principles of State Policy (DPSP) and are not justifiable. Under the DPSP, Articles 38,[2] 39 and 47 deal with the duties of the state to provide better health to its citizens (Desai et al., 2007). The Constitution has made health care services largely the state's responsibility but left enough space for the centre since many items are listed in the concurrent list.[3]

With the dissolution of the Indian Medical Service, farewell of a number of British doctors and the paucity of indigenous health care professionals after independence led to a huge rift in public health services (Borkar, 1961). To fill this gap, we obtained a health policy document, but it took 35 years after independence for the government to make a health policy statement in 1982–83. And it is no coincidence that such a policy statement came only after the 1978 Alma Ata Declaration[4] of the World Health Assembly—Health for All by 2000 AD. But this does not mean that there was no health policy all these years. There was a distinct policy and strategy for the health sector, albeit an unwritten one. This was reflected through the different Five-Year Plans.

MATERNAL AND CHILD HEALTH AND FIVE-YEAR PLANS

India witnessed the emergence of various Government Committees constituted by the central government over the years to look at the challenges in the health sector and to give recommendations for overcoming them. On the basis of the recommendations and suggestions, different programmes and policies were framed through Five-Year plans, which give us a picture of the efforts taken by India in the development of health of its citizens. Different initiatives were taken with respect to the mother and child health rights from the initiation itself.

The National Planning Committee, appointed in 1938, began its work early in 1939 under the aegis of Col. S.S. Sokhey. The Committee was divided into 29 sub-committees, formed into eight groups to deal with all dynamics of health, life and work with a predetermined plan. After some unavoidable delays, the report was submitted in 1940. Towards the end of the year, the Chairman, Pandit Jawaharlal Nehru, was arrested and sentenced to a long-term imprisonment and the war with Japan also broke out. These two reasons put the activity of some sub-committees into cold storage. Its report, published in 1948, was sketchy and it was not studied as well, and it lacked in detailed analysis of the existing health situation as well as of the future plans. In fact, it borrowed its analysis of the health situation from another committee, that is, the Bhore Committee, and also concurred with most of its recommendations (NPC, 1948). One of the members of the sub-committee looking over the health dimension was Ms Rani Laxshmibai Rajwade, who was looking at the different aspects of Maternal and Child Welfare Services. In her report, she tried to paint the grim picture of maternal and child mortality and suggested many useful recommendations. In her report, she claimed that maternal and Child Welfare being a basic health service might well be thought to have a primary claim on public funds, but unfortunately the aims and objects of the movement are somewhat imperfectly understood and the potential benefits to the health of the community are not sufficiently appreciated. In consequence, the expenditure of public funds on maternity and child welfare is still very limited.

She also recommended in her report the need for a central statutory body. This great social cause has not made much headway in India chiefly because there has been no recognition so far of its fundamental importance and urgency. The total effort being mainly voluntary and local so far has had behind it neither the resources nor the authority nor the co-ordination, unity and drive which are its due.

She also quoted from the Report of the Director of Public Health, Bengal, 1947, that 'The maternity and child welfare work is mainly a responsibility of the local bodies....'

Thus, it stated and emphasized the necessity for a permanent central body for the protection of motherhood and childhood under the Ministry of Health having a major portion of the resources allocated, and every state should have its own department or institute for the protection of motherhood and childhood.

Another development was the Health Survey and Development Committee popularly known as 'Bhore Committee', appointed by the Government of India under the chairmanship of Sir Joseph Bhore on 18 October 1943, with an object to make a survey on the existing health conditions and make recommendations for future development. Its secretary was Dr K.C.K.E. Raja and one of the joint secretaries was Dr K.T. Jungalwala. Some of the well-known members included Dr J.B. Grant, Dr B.C. Roy, Pandit P.N. Sapru and Dr A.L. Mudaliar. This Committee prepared a detailed plan of a National Health Service for the country, which would provide a universal coverage to the entire population, free of charges through a comprehensive state-run, salaried health service. Such a well-studied and minutely documented plan has not yet been prepared in independent India.

In 1949, 'Dasgupta Committee', also known as Environmental Hygiene Committee, was appointed under the chairmanship of Dr B.C. Dasgupta who was also a member of Bhore Committee, with an objective of looking into housing, water supply, general sanitation and drainage systems, waste disposal, vector control, etc., which indirectly affects the health of mother and child. In 1955, 'Model Public Health Act Committee' was established to bring all health legislation under one umbrella and rationalizing them (Table 5.2).

In 1951, our infant democracy took stock of the existing situation in the country and initiated the First Five-Year Development Plan. Living in a resource-poor country with high population density, the planners recognized in the census figures of 1951, the potential threat posed by population explosion and the need to take steps to avert it. It was recognized that population stabilization is an essential prerequisite for sustainability of development process so that the benefits of economic development result in enhancement of the well-being of the people and improvement in the quality of life (GoI, 1951). India is the first country in the world to formulate a National Family Planning Programme in 1952, with the objective of 'reducing birth rate to the extent necessary to stabilize the population at a level consistent with requirement of national economy'. Thus, the

Table 5.2 Major Health Committees Related to MCH Constituted by the Government of India

Year	*Name of the Committee*
1940	Sokhey Committee (Sub-Committee of the National Planning Committee)
1946	Bhore Committee
1949	Dasgupta Committee
1955	Model Public Health Act Committee
1961	Mudaliar Committee
1963	Chadah Committee
1964	Ayyar Committee
1966	Mukharjee Committee
1966	Shah Committee
1967	Jungalwala Committee
1973	Kartar Singh Committee
1975	Shrivastava Committee
1975	Hathi Committee
1978	Small Family Norm Committee
1981	ICSSR and ICMR Study Group[5]
1987	Bajaj Committee

key elements of health care to women and children and provision of contraceptive services have been the focus of India's health services right from the time of India's independence (WHO, 1952). The first two Five-Year Plans (1951–61) made their allocations to implement the Bhore Committee recommendations, especially related to building up a primary bedrock for health services in the country. The policy and strategies address the MCH in an integrated fashion. To prevent diseases relating to nutritional deficiency, school-feeding programmes were recommended. Malaria and tuberculosis received primary importance in the disease control programme. An MCH training centre was also established at the All India Institute of Hygiene and Public Health with the aim of assisting the United Nations International Children's Emergency Fund (UNICEF).[6] A total of 200 MCH centres were established in different states during the period of

First Five-Year Plan (Basavanthappa, 2008). The Central Government constituted the 'Mudaliar Committee' in June 1959 to review the First and Second Five-Year Plans (1951–61) health projects. The Mudaliar Committee in 1962 recommended, for instance, the expansion of MCH centres to include one ANM per 10,000 population (GoI, 1962).

On the basis of the recommendations of Mudaliar Committee, special attention was given to MCH. The states were provided nearly ₹ 3 crores for setting up about 2,100 maternity and child health centres. These centres were directed to be integrated with the primary health unit services. The need for proper training of medical and ancillary personnel to be employed in maternal and child health programmes was recognized and the plan makes the necessary provision. Paediatric training was also provided to personnel who were in charge of maternal and child health centres in the paediatric departments of medical colleges and to equip them suitably.

Table 5.3 depicts the Human Resource for Health from 1950 to 1960 and the existing gap. By the end of the Second Plan, Human Resource for Health (HRH) was increased substantially but not up to the requirement, especially HRH directly relating to MCH programmes.

Shortages in personnel other than doctors had been marked. At the end of 1954, the numbers registered in different categories in the states were 20,793 nurses, 24,290 midwives, 756 health visitors, 4,468 *Dais* and 946 nurse *Dais*. As norms to aim at, there should be one hospital bed for 1,000 population, one nurse and one midwife for every 5,000 population and one health visitor and one sanitary inspector

Table 5.3 Existing Human Resource for Health and the Gap

	1950–51	*1955–56*	*1960–61*	*As per norms*
Doctors	59,000	70,000	82,500	90,000
Nurses (including auxiliary nurse midwives or ANMs)	17,000	22,000	31,000	80,000
Midwives	18,000	26,000	32,000	80,000
Health visitors	600	800	2500	20,000
Nurse *Dais*	4,000	6,000	41,000	80,000

per 20,000 population. It is worthwhile noting that the basis on which the total number of midwives was estimated by the Bhore Committee was one midwife for a total of 100 births per year. For 10 million births per year, they estimated a total requirement of 100,000 midwives—the goal that appeared a distant dream to be achieved (GoI, 1956).

At the end of Second Plan, the number of primary health units increased to 2,800 as against 725 units during the First-Plan period. Also, there was 4,500 maternity and child welfare centres across the country during this period (ibid.). But the presence of female doctors at the Primary Health Centre (PHC) level was exceptional. Only 15 per cent of the total PHCs had the minimum requirement of two doctors. At the end of the Second Plan, an important act, that is, The Maternity Benefit Act, 1961, was also enacted, which strengthened the MCH concept in India (MoHFW, 1961).

What was even more significant was that, instead of expanding this bedrock of health services further, the Mudaliar Committee in 1962 recommended for strengthening the existing PHCs. Its logic was that the HRH of the existing PHCs was inadequately skilled and was not oriented to maternity care. In place of expanding training programmes or reorientation of medical education, the Mudaliar Committee suggested consolidation of existing PHCs with a larger number of doctors and public health nurses. It also proposed mobile dispensaries for proper networking of rural population and health service delivery system. Over and above this, it also recommended to establish specialist services including paediatric and maternity hospitals in urban areas.

Accepting a few recommendations and rejecting the others, a sharp shift took place at the policy level in favour of urban areas at the cost of rural areas. The Third Five-Year Plan (1961–66) reflected this trend, that is, specialization and hospitals acquired priority over training of HRH and creation of PHCs and sub-centres (GoI, 1961). Maternity and child services were also overshadowed by these trends. The most dominating actors during the plan were National Malaria Eradication Programme and the Family Planning Programme and even the name of the chapter in the Plan documents was changed from 'Health' to 'Health and Family Planning'. Thus, the share of health in the total outlay was reduced from 5.6 per cent in the Second Plan to 5 and 4 per cent in the Third and Fourth Plans, respectively (see Table 5.4). Even within the health sector allocation, malaria got the largest piece of the cake; thus, maternity services bore the brunt of this decreased resource.

Table 5.4 Five-Year Plans Outlay and Pattern of Allocation

Period	*Total Plan Allocation*	*Health*	*%*	*Family Welfare*	*%*
First Plan (1951–56)	1960.00	65.20	3.33	0.10	0.01
Second Plan (1956–61)	4672	140.80	3.01	5.00	0.11
Third Plan (1961–66)	8576.50	225.90	2.63	24.90	0.29
Fourth Plan (1969–74)	15,778.80	335.50	2.13	278.00	1.76
Fifth Plan (1974–79)	39,426.20	760.80	1.93	491.80	1.25

The Malaria Eradication Programme reached its maturity in India after 1960 and the 'Chadha Committee' of 1962 was constituted to evaluate the programme. The Committee recommended that all the basic health workers would function as multipurpose workers, in addition to their malaria works and carry out the duties of family planning and collating vital statistics, thus health and family planning services were integrated.

Family Planning Programmes (FPPs) initially followed clinical approach, but after the 1962 census, which showed continuous rise in population growth of 21.5 per cent, the central government decided to adopt demographic goal to reach a crude birth rate of 25 by the year 1972. In 1965, the 'Mukherjee Committee' was formed to review staffing pattern and financial provision under FPP (MoHFW, 1968). The Committee found that the recommendations of the Chadha Committee could not be implemented, because basic health workers could do justice to neither malaria programme nor family planning work. Therefore, the recommendation was to bifurcate the two responsibilities, with family planning assistants looking after family planning work; thus, a separate department for family planning was constituted at the centre during 1966. The other factor that paved the way for the establishment of the centre was the international pressure from various developed countries. In 1966, a UN Advisory Mission visiting India strongly recommended that the directorate (health and family planning) should be relieved from other responsibilities such as maternal and child health and nutrition. It is undoubtedly important for family planning to be integrated with MCH in the field particularly in view of the loop programme, but until the family planning campaign has picked up momentum and made real progress in the states, the director general concerned should be responsible for family planning only. (U.N. Advisory Mission 1961)

As a result, a vertical FPP treated maternity services as a *pariah* and left it untouched but not for too long. Because of the close linkages between the two, and with a view to give broader base to the FPP, it was decided in 1967 that MCH be integrated with FPP (Pandey et al., 2004). With the integration of FPP, new programmes for MCH were introduced with a tag of neo-Malthusian, for example, the Postpartum Programme introduced in 1969 for the women coming for deliveries, with an eye to enhance acceptance of female sterilization. Another example is of Intensive District Programmes initiated to cover the most populous states. Thus, FPP starting with clinical approach shifted to extension, followed by targets and later compulsion approaches and ultimately transformed into family welfare programme.

The trend of integrating specific initiatives into larger and more comprehensive programmes began with the Fourth Plan. The Plan began in 1969 with a three-year plan holiday. MCH services were integrated and an integrated nutrition programme was proposed. In addition, a new scheme for preschool children in the form of *Balwardis* was initiated. It lamented on the poor progress made in the PHC programme and recognized again the need to strengthen it. It pleaded for the establishment of effective machinery for speedy construction of buildings and improvement of the performance of PHCs by providing them with staff, equipment and other facilities. In 1970–71, the social welfare department also started special feeding programmes for children below the age of three years in tribal areas and urban slums. Further, this programme was extended to children up to six years, pregnant women and lactating mothers (GoI, 1969).

However, the Plan continued on the same line as the Third Plan. It quoted extensively from the Second Five-Year Plan. In fact, the Fourth Plan is probably the most poorly written plan document. It does not even make a passing comment on the social, political and economic upheaval during the Plan Holiday Period (1966–69). These three years of turmoil indeed brought about significant policy changes on the economic front and, thus, the Fourth Plan was ignored completely.

In the dismal scenario of growth, where maternity services were completely overshadowed by the FPP, the Fifth Five-Year Plan (1974–79) did make an effort to integrate FPP, MCH and nutrition services and highlighted the problems of malnutrition and anaemia and their implications for MCH (GoI, 1974). The importance of primary health care to the rural population was again recognized during the Plan period with the Minimum Need Programme. The plan period also saw the launch of the Integrated Child Development Services (ICDSs) scheme in 1975 and adoption of 'National Policy for Children' in 1977, which directs the state to provide adequate services to children, both before and after birth and through the period of growth to ensure their full physical, mental and social development. This provision further strengthened the MCH movement in India. Thus, at the end of the Plan, maternal health was seen as an essential component of child development, and hence, pre- and post-natal services were included in the different initiatives (Debroy and Mahal, 2010).

The 'Kartar Singh Committee' in 1973 recommended the conversion of uni-purpose workers, including ANMs, into multipurpose male and female workers and existence of one PHC for a population of 50,000. The Committee recommended that each pair of such workers should serve a population of 10,000–12,000. Hence, the multipurpose worker scheme was launched with the objective to retrain the existing cadre of vertical programme workers, and the various vertical programmes were to be fully integrated into the primary health care package for rural areas. Another major innovation in the health strategy was launched in 1977 by creating a cadre of village-based health auxiliaries, called the community health workers. These were part-time workers selected by the village and trained for three months in simple promotive and curative skills in both allopathy and indigenous systems of medicine. They were to be supervised by multipurpose workers (MPWs), and the programme was started in 777 selected PHCs where MPWs were already in place. This scheme was adopted on the recommendations of the 'Shrivastava Committee' (Shrivastava, 1975), which was essentially a committee to look into medical education and support manpower. In the same year, another committee known as 'Hathi Committee' was formed with the objective of addressing the issue by increasing the prices of life-saving and other drugs and dependence on multinational companies for drug availability.

The Plan was, however, prematurely terminated due to declaration of national emergency. During this period, the Ministry of Health and Family Planning opted for compulsory sterilization, which led to a major political debate and debacle.

The Sixth Plan was to a great extent influenced by the Alma Ata Declaration of Health for All by 2000 AD and the ICSSR–ICMR Report (1980). The plan conceded that 'there is a serious dissatisfaction with the existing model of medical and health services with its emphasis on hospitals, specialization and super-specialization and highly trained doctors, which is availed of mostly by the well-to-do classes. It is also realized that it is this model which is depriving the rural areas and the poor people of the benefits of good health and medical services.' The plan emphasized the development of a community-based health system. The plan emphasized that horizontal and vertical linkages had to be established among all the interrelated programmes, such as water supply, environmental sanitation, hygiene, nutrition, education, family planning and MCH. The objective of achieving a net reproduction rate of one by 1995 (GoI, 1981) was reiterated. This plan and the seventh plan too, like the earlier ones, make a lot of radical statements and have recommended progressive measures. But the story is the same—progressive thinking and inadequate action. However, the Sixth and the Seventh Plans are different from the earlier ones in one respect. They no longer talk of targets. The National Health Policy of 1983 was announced during the Sixth-Plan period.

After the implementation of the Seventh Plan (1984–89), the family welfare programme evolved with a dual force: first, on the health needs of women in the reproductive age group and of children below the age of five years, and second, to provide contraceptives and family planning services (GoI, 1985). The Universal Immunization Programme and Oral Rehydration Therapy (ORT) were initiated to curb down the mortality and morbidity among infants and young children (Debroy and Mahal, 2010).

On the eve of the Eighth Five-Year Plan (1992–97), the country went through a massive economic crisis. The Plan got pushed forward by two years. But despite this, no new thinking went into this plan. In fact, keeping with the selective health care approach, the Eighth Plan adopted a new slogan—instead of Health for All by 2000 AD, it chose to emphasize Health for the Underprivileged (GoI, 1992). The Plan emphasized a community-based system covering about 3,000 people as the basic unit of the primary health care system.

During the Eighth Plan, resources were provided to set up the Education Commission for Health Sciences, and a few states have even set up the University for Health Sciences as per the recommendations of the Bajaj Committee Report of 1987. The first phase of Reproductive and Child Health (RCH) Programme was also launched in 1997 by integrating all ongoing fertility regulation and MCH schemes of the Ministry under a single umbrella, adopting a holistic target-free approach. It was flagship programme of family welfare, which combines the trinity of objectives, that is, reproductive health, child survival and fertility regulations with a policy and a programme orientation. The overall goals of the programme were to reduce maternal and infant mortality and morbidity and give a sure reproductive health choice (Mavalankar, 2011).

The National Maternity Benefit Scheme (NMBS) was also launched on 15 August 1995, aiming to provide maternal care in the form of better diet to expectant mothers. This scheme provided financial assistance of ₹ 500 per birth for the first two births to all the pregnant women who attained 19 years of age and belonged to Below Poverty Line (BPL) households (MoHFW, 1996).

During the Eighth-Plan period, a committee to review public health was set up. It was called the Expert Committee on Public Health Systems. This committee made a thorough appraisal of public health programmes and found that we were facing a resurgence of most communicable diseases, and there was a need to drastically improve disease surveillance in the country. The Ninth Plan proposed to set up, at district level, a strong detection-cum-response system for rapid containment of any outbreaks that may occur. In fact, the recommendations of this committee have formed the basis of the Ninth Plan health sector strategy to revitalize the public health system in the country to respond to its health care needs in these changed times. Also, the Plan has proposed horizontal integration of all vertical programmes at the district level to increase their effectiveness as also to facilitate allocative efficiencies (GoI, 1997). What was also interesting was that the Ninth Plan also reviewed the National Health Policy, 1983.

The Ninth Plan also reviews population policy and the family planning programme. In this review too, it goes back to the Bhore Committee Report and says that the core of this programme is MCH services. Assuring antenatal care (ANC), safe delivery and immunization are critical to reducing infant and maternal mortality, and this, in turn, has bearing on contraception use and fertility rates. This is old logic, which the family planning programme has used, only earlier their emphasis was on sterilization. In the early sixties, the setting up of sub-centres and employing ANMs was precisely for the MCH programme; but at the field level, this was hijacked by the family planning programme. This story continues through the 1970s and 1980s. MCH became Safe Motherhood and expanded Programme of Immunization, and the latter using a mission approach under Sam Pitroda became Universal Programme of Immunization. In the Seventh Plan, this got combined again to become Child Survival and Safe Motherhood (CSSM), but the essential emphasis remained on family planning. But since the Eighth Plan and in the Ninth Plan, CSSM acquired a genuine seriousness. In the midst of all this, the National Population Policy was announced with a lot of fanfare in the mid-2000. It is definitely an improvement of its predecessors, but the underlying element remains population control and not population welfare. From this plan onwards, allocation was done separately for Health and Family welfare instead of under Social Service Sector.

The Tenth-Plan period (2002–07) witnessed a transition in health care policies and strategies with the effecting of an architectural correction in the health care delivery system at the primary and secondary levels and the steps taken to set in motion regional balance in the availability of tertiary health care facilities. Wide-ranging reforms and policy initiatives have been taken for improving health infrastructure and addressing the health care needs of the population. Several initiatives have also been undertaken on the disease front to curtail morbidity and mortality. A National Health Policy was also formulated during the year 2002 that highlighted 14 goals to be achieved within the time frame and welcomed private participation in all areas of health activities (GoI, 2002). Other major committees in this period include the Mashelkar Committee in Drug Regulatory Issues, 2003, and the National Commission on Macro Economics and Health, 2005.

India is committed to achieving the MDGs set by UN MDGs set by the UN Millennium Declaration 2000. As a result, they have been incorporated smoothly into the Eleventh Five-Year Plan (2007–12). The plan also acknowledges the need for action on many fronts such as improved access to health centres, institutional deliveries, nutritional supplementation, and clean drinking water and sanitation. The Plan positions the development of children at its centre and recognizes nutrition as critical for ensuring child survival and development. It accords high priority to addressing maternal and child under nutrition through multi-sectoral interventions by different sectors (GoI, 2007).

On the basis of key learning of the first RCH programme and to reduce the gap and lacuna, the RCH-II was launched on 1 April 2005, under the aegis of National Rural Health Mission (NRHM). The main objective was to bring about a change in three critical health indicators, that is, total fertility rate, infant mortality rate (IMR) and maternal mortality rate (MMR). The maternal health programme that is a component of the RCH programme aims at reducing maternal mortality to less than 150 by 2010 through a number of interventions to curb the major causes of these deaths such as haemorrhage (both ante- and postpartum), toxaemia (hypertension during pregnancy), anaemia, obstructed labour, puerperal sepsis (infections after delivery) and unsafe abortion. The interventions were providing essential obstetric care, at least three antenatal check-ups for tracking preventive and promotive steps and to detect complications early for prompt action and at least three post-natal check-ups to monitor the post-natal recovery (Bhat, 1993; Bose, 2001).

Another flagship scheme launched in the plan period was *Janani Suraksha Yojana* (JSY). With a little modification in NMBS, JSY centrally sponsored scheme was launched on 12 April 2005 and implemented in all states and union territories (UTs). It is a safe motherhood intervention under the umbrella of NRHM with an objective of reducing maternal and neonatal mortality by promoting institutional delivery among the poor pregnant women belonging to the BPL households and of the age 19 years or above for up to two live births. The *Yojana* has identified the accredited social health activist (ASHA) as an effective link between the government and the poor pregnant women in 10 low-performing states namely eight Empowered Action Group[7] states and Assam and Jammu and Kashmir, the remaining North East States and tribal districts of all other states. Her main role is to facilitate pregnant women to avail services of maternal care and arrange referral transport.

Regarding forthcoming Twelfth Five-Year Plan, Sayeeda Hameed, member of the Planning Commission said in a press interview that MCH is expected to be the thrust area in the Twelfth Five-Year Plan (2012–17).

Table 5.5 Five-Year Plans Outlay and Pattern of Allocation (Continued from Table 5.4)

Period	*Total Plan Allocation*	*Health*	*%*	*Family Welfare*	*%*
Annual Plans	12,176.5	223.1	1.8	118.5	1
Sixth Plan	97,500	1821	1.9	1010	1
Seventh Plan	180,000	3392.9	1.9	3256.3	1.8
Annual Plans	127,373.9	2003.2	1.6	1641.5	1.3
Eight Plan	434,100	7494.2	1.7	6500	1.5
Ninth Plan	859,200	19,818.4	2.3	15,120.2	1.8
Tenth Plan	1,484,131.3	31,020.3	2.1	27,125	1.8
Eleventh Plan	2,156,571	41,092.9	1.9	90,558	4.2

From the 1950–2007 Five Year-Plans period, the percentage of total health sector outlay in the total planned investment in the country was almost stagnant or even fell during some plan periods (see Tables 5.4 and 5.5). Moreover, there was a decreasing trend in the allocation under the head 'Health' as a percentage of total planned investment. However, in the case of 'Family Welfare', its share increased.

MATERNAL AND CHILD HEALTH AND HEALTH POLICIES IN INDIA

Health policy of a nation is its strategy for controlling and optimizing the social uses of its health knowledge and health resources. At the turn of the twenty-first century, India acquired two new policies, one for health and the other for population. India had its first national health policy in 1983, that is, 36 years after independence. The seed of this plan was sown in the joint WHO-UNICEF International Conference in 1978 at Alma-Ata (USSR) known as the Alma-Ata Conference (Mavalankar, 2011).

National Health Policy, 1983

Alma-Ata Declaration called on all the governments to formulate national health policies according to their own circumstances to launch and sustain primary health care as a part of national health system. Thus, the Indian government came up with the National Health Policy in the light of the Directive Principles of the Constitution of

India, which recommends 'universal, comprehensive primary health care services which are relevant to the actual needs and priorities of the community at a cost which people can afford' (MoHFW, 1983). Providing universal health care as a goal is a welcome step because this is the first time after the Bhore Committee that the government is talking of universal comprehensive health care.

National Health Policy (NHP) 1983 was based on four principles. First, there would have to be a time-bound programme for setting up a comprehensive network of primary health services with health education. Second, intermediation would be pushed through health volunteers who would have the requisite knowledge and skills and access to necessary technologies. Third, there would be a well-organized referral system, so that medical personnel at higher levels of care would not be burdened with patients who could be treated by first-level providers. Fourth, there would be an integrated network of speciality and super-speciality services and the setting of these facilities would be encouraged through private partnership. The policy stressed the need for providing primary health care with special emphasis on prevention, promotion and rehabilitation and suggested planned time-bound attention to the following:

1. Nutrition, prevention of food adulteration
2. Maintenance of quality of drugs
3. Water supply and sanitation
4. Environmental protection
5. Immunization programme
6. Maternal and child health services
7. School health programme
8. Occupational health services

For a better programme planning, NHP 1983, recommended an effective Health Information System and to achieve a target of IMR of 60 and MMR of 200 by 2000 as was given in Alma Ata Declaration. During the decade following the NHP 1983, rural health care received special attention and a massive programme of expansion of primary health care facilities was undertaken in the Sixth and Seventh Five-Year Plans to achieve the target of one PHC per 30,000 population and one sub-centre per 5,000 population. However, the financial resources and public health administrative capacity was far short of that necessary to achieve such an ambitious and holistic goal. The target has more or less been achieved, although few states still lagged behind.

National Health Policy, 2002

The second major policy endeavour is the National Health Policy, 2002, and it closely followed on the heels of the National Population Policy, 2000. Both policies grew in the context of liberalization and globalization. The concept of Health for All and Health is a Fundamental Human Right, which was the cornerstone of the Soviet Health Policy, was given a goodbye in this policy. After the collapse of the Soviet Union, the health programmes were also gradually privatized. The focus of the policy ought to be on reforming the public health system. Moreover, it focused urban centric, specialist-based health care by ignoring the pressing needs of primary health care services. It proposed privatization of secondary- and tertiary-level care, ignoring the fact that 45 per cent of the poorest in the country depends on public hospitals for critical indoor care (Qadeer, 2011). Another loophole of the policy was the provision of user fees in public hospitals. However, ambitious health goals were set in NHP 2002.

It was followed by a massive NRHM, launched by the Prime Minister in 2005.

National Rural Health Mission, 2005

The NRHM, launched in 2005 with a seven-year mandate, subsumed within its programmes, aimed at reproductive and child health, killer diseases, deficiency diseases, etc. The NRHM is the key plank for giving effect to the mandate of the National Common Minimum Programme (NCMP). The NRHM also provides an overarching umbrella to the existing programmes of Health and Family Welfare including RCH-II, etc. The objective of the NRHM is to improve the availability of, and access to, quality health care, especially for those living in rural areas, the poor, women and children. The core strategies of the mission include identification and selection of the ASHA, decentralized planning, strengthening of existing infrastructure such as sub-centres, PHCs and CHCs, adoption of sectorwide approach, community participation, manpower development, and partnership with non-governmental stakeholders. MCH was the basic thrust and always kept on the front seat of the programme (NRHM, 2005).

One of the prime actors in the Mission is the ASHA, the woman responsible for a variety of tasks, but she does not have a fixed remuneration. The group dealing with strengthening community health care recommended that there should be one ASHA for every 1,000 population; however, in tribal, hilly and desert areas, there should be one ASHA per habitation. She must be an 'ever-married' woman volunteer in the 25–45 age group and from a disadvantaged group. Literacy as an eligibility criterion should not be a limiting condition.

But the Mission document is silent on these aspects. Neither does it specify the population covered by the ASHA nor the professional cadres who would be supervising their working. The ASHA will be an honorary volunteer. She would act as a bridge between the ANM and the village, accountable to the village *panchayat* and an important link worker in JSY.

The NRHM had injected new hope into the health care delivery system in India. However, it faced diverse challenges, which need to be focused if its goals are to be achieved in the near future. The first hurdle is the location of health in the State List rather than the Concurrent List posing major problems for service delivery (*The Hindu*, 2012). This was also compounded by the fact that the NRHM funding was from the Centre while the implementation was by the state governments. The next problem is related to the nature of the NRHM. It was in a shape of project which ended in April, 2012, and if its funding will be ceased/reduced in the Twelfth Five-Year Plan, then a rift will be formed in the country's health status. The third problem is its target population. The NRHM had focused on rural health, neglecting the health needs of women and children of urban India. The scams related to the fund transfer and purchasing of medicines and equipments affected the quality of services delivered under NRHM (Jacob, 2011).

Health care delivery cannot be improved to provide a seamless service without the removal of these barriers. The NRHM added new infrastructure and personnel; however, its impact on re-inventing and re-invigorating systems seems to be limited with much more efforts being required (Bajpai et al., 2010). There is a need for a more coordinated approach that optimally utilizes resources.

MATERNAL AND CHILD HEALTH AND RELIABLE INFORMATION SYSTEM IN INDIA

Reliable national estimates of maternal mortality are not available for most countries since most of the demographic surveys do not have samples large enough to produce reliable direct estimates of maternal mortality. In India, different organizations are involved in researching different dimensions of health and giving us the correct picture at macro- and micro-levels.

National Family Health Survey (NFHS) and Sample Registration System (SRS) are the two important Indian health information systems in providing information on different health indicators at macro level, covering fertility and family planning, mortality and morbidity, health, health care and nutrition and also prevalence of HIV/AIDs. A major objective of the NFHS under the aegis of Indian Institute of Population Sciences (IIPS) was to provide information on MCH practices. The relevant information was collected in the Women's Questionnaire from the mothers of all children born since 1 January 1988 for states where the NFHS was initiated in 1992 and 1 January 1989, where the NFHS was carried out in 1993. The information covered matters related to pregnancy and childbirth, ANC infant and child-feeding practices, including breastfeeding, immunizations, episodes of illness such as acute respiratory infection, fever and diarrhoea, and the treatment received, mother's knowledge and use of oral rehydration salts (ORS), and the level of child nutrition assessed by measuring the weight and height of children. The first round of NFHS was conducted in 1992–93, and the second round was conducted during 1998–99. The current survey of NFHS was undertaken during 2005–06 covering 1.1 lakh households and interviewing about 2.3 lakh eligible men and women. The NFHS-1 provided a national estimate of 424 in 1992–93. The NFHS-2 suggested that the MMR had not changed significantly from 424 in 1992–93 to 540 in 1998–99. However, the figure was reduced to 230 in 2005–06.

SRS managed by the Registrar General of India is an annual survey started in 1970, which provides estimated parameters on fertility and mortality indicators at the macro level.

Since the indicators estimated through SRS and NFHS are confined to state level only, the concept of providing similar indicators at district level had been perceived through District-Level Household Surveys (DLHS). The first round of DLHS was undertaken in 1998–99, the second DLHS was undertaken during 2002–04, followed by the third one in 2006–07 at an interval of four years.

CONCLUDING NOTE

Women are the half of human wealth of India and today's children are tomorrow's healthy India. The health of both, that is, women and children matters a lot for building healthy India. Right after the Independence, under the Eleventh Five-Year Plans and three National Health Policies, central as well as state authorities had taken different steps, initiated projects, trained personnel and undertook health programmes for mothers and children. The result of the meticulous planning and policies could be realized from the improvement in the various health indicators.

Considerable achievements have been made over the past six decades in our efforts to improve health standards, such as fertility rate, IMR and MMR. But still, India remains one of the unhealthiest countries of the world and painting an unimpressive picture in respect of all health indicators.

To sum up, we need to restructure the overall policies and programmes for achieving a new vision-based, broad-based and inclusive growth at faster rate. Budgets for health services will need to increase by a factor of three or five times. Every effort must be made to achieve good health for people, especially the poor and underprivileged women and children.

NOTES

1. An incantation in Sanskrit taken from Taittirīya Upanishad, which makes the mother as the first among gods and goddesses.
2. Article 38 of the Indian Constitution urges the State to secure a social order for the promotion of welfare of people. Article 39 contains certain principles to be followed by the State for securing health and strength of workers, men and women and more specifically to protect the freedom and dignity of childhood and youth. Article 47 states that the State shall regard the raising of the level of nutrition and the standard of living of its people and the improvement of public health as among its primary duties.
3. According to the Indian Constitution, all activities of the government are categorized into three: Central List, State List and Concurrent List. Activities that fall under the Concurrent List are mostly subject to overlapping jurisdiction between the central and state governments.
4. The Alma Ata Declaration was adopted at the International Conference on Primary Health Care, Alma Ata (in the former USSR).
5. This group was set up after India became signatory to the Alma Ata Declaration of Health for All by 2000 AD.
6. Now known as United Nations Children's Fund.
7. The Empowered Action Group (EAG) states are those with high fertility rates and weak socio-demographic indicators (Hindi belt states).

REFERENCES

Bajpai, N., J.D. Sachs and R.H. Dholakia, 2010, *Improving Access and Efficiency in Public Health Services*. New Delhi: Sage Publication.

Basavanthappa, B.T., 2008, *Community Health Nursing*, 2nd ed. New Delhi: Jaypee Publishers.

Bhat, M., 1993, 'Maternal Mortality and MCH Services', *Economic and Poilitical Weekly*, March 6, XXVIII(10): 362.

Bhore, S.J., 1946, *Report of the Health Survey and Development Committee*. Calcutta: Government of India Press.

Borkar, G., 1961, *Health in Independent India*. New Delhi: Ministry of Health, Government of India.

Bose, A., 2001, 'Health For All: Broken Promises', *Economic and Political Weekly*, 36(11): 905–07.

Debroy, B. and A. Mahal, 2010, 'Health Reform: A Historical Perspective and the Future'. In *India Health Report 2010*, edited by A. Mahal, B. Debroy and L. Bhandari, New Delhi: Indicus Analytics, pp. 127–35.

Desai, M. and D. Chand, 2007, 'Fundamental Right to Health and Public Health Care'. In *Health Care Case Law in India: A Reader*, edited by M. Desai and K.B. Mahabal, New Delhi: CEHAT & ICHRL, pp. 17–35.

Government of India (GoI), 1951, *First Five-Year Plan*. New Delhi: Planning Commission.

Government of India (GoI), 1956, *Second Five-Year Plan*. New Delhi: Planning Commission.

Government of India (GoI), 1961, *Third Five-Year Plan*. New Delhi: Planning Commission.

Government of India (GoI), 1962, *Report of the Health Survey and Planning Committee (Mudaliar Committee)*. New Delhi: Planning Commission.

Government of India (GoI), 1969, *Fourth Five-Year Plan*. New Delhi: Planning Commission.

Government of India (GoI), 1974, *Fifth Five-Year Plan*. New Delhi: Planning Commission.

Government of India (GoI), 1981, *Sixth Five-Year Plan*. New Delhi: Planning Commission.

Government of India (GoI), 1985, *Seventh Five-Year Plan*. New Delhi: Planning Commission.

Government of India (GoI), 1992, *Eight Five-Year Plan*. New Delhi: Planning Commission.

Government of India (GoI), 1997, *Ninth Five-Year Plan*. New Delhi: Planning Commission.

Government of India (GoI), 2002, *Tenth Five-Year Plan*. New Delhi: Planning Commission.

Government of India (GoI), 2007, *Draft Report on Recommendation of Task Force on Public Private Partnership for the 11th Plan*. New Delhi: Planning Commission.

Government of India (GoI), 2007, *Eleventh Five-Year Plan*. New Delhi: Planning Commission.

Jacob, K.S., 2011, 'For a New and Improved NRHM', *The Hindu*, August 8: 10.

Jeffrey, R., 1988, *Politics of Health in India*. Berkeley: University of California.

Mavalankar, D., 2011, 'Universal Health Care: The Barriers and the Way Forward', *The Hindu*, July 6.

Ministry of Health and Family Welfare, Government of India (MoHFW), 1961, *Report of the Health Survey and Planning Committee*.

Ministry of Health and Family Welfare, Government of India (MoHFW), 1968, *Mukherjee Committee Report: Part II*.

Ministry of Health and Family Welfare, Government of India (MoHFW), 1983, *National Health Policy*.

Ministry of Health and Family Welfare, Government of India (MoHFW), 1996, *Report of the Expert Committee on Public Health System*.

Ministry of Health and Family Welfare, Government of India (MoHFW), *First Five Year Plan Document*.

National Planning Committee, 1948, *Report on Sub-Committee on National Health (Sokhey Committee)*. Bombay: Vora & Co.

NRHM, 2005, *National Rural Health Mission 2005–2012: Mission Document*. New Delhi: Ministry of Health anf Family Welfare.

Pandey, A., N. Roy, D. Sahu and R. Acharya, 2004, 'Maternal Health Care Services', *Economic and Political Weekly*, February 14.

Qadeer, I., 2011, *Public Health in India: Critical Reflections*. New Delhi: Danish Books.

Shah, K.T., 1948, *National Health (Report of the Sub-Committee)*. Bombay: Vora & Co., Publishers Ltd.

Shrivastava, J.B. 1975, *Health Services and Medical Education: A Programme for Immediate Action*. New Delhi: Allied Publishers.

The Hindu, 2012, 'Searches on, New Cases Filed in U.P. NRHM Scam', February 25.

World Health Organisation, 1952, *Expert Committee on Maternity Care: First Report – A Preliminary Survey*. Geneva: WHO.

Part II

Reproductive Trajectory: From Pregnancy to Childbirth

CHAPTER 6

Culture, Social Class, Technology and Pain: A Sociological Analysis of Pain in Childbirth

Sayantika Palit

INTRODUCTION

The history of childbirth, especially in the context of the United States, can be divided into three periods. Until the late eighteenth century, birth was exclusively a female affair, a social event managed by midwives and relatives. The second period, from the late eighteenth to the first decades of the twentieth century, was a long transition between social childbirth and medical birth. With time, male physicians replaced midwives and transformed birth into a medical event. The biomedical model of birth emerged with the Industrial Revolution; and by the 1920s, it had consolidated its position (Dye, 1980).

The question that we may ask is: Why did women turn to physicians? Some scholars argue that it is due to the promise of safer, less painful labour through the use of forceps, drugs and anaesthesia. Increasing knowledge of the physiology of labour, ability to handle difficult labours with forceps and surgery promised greater safety (ibid.).

As the medical control got consolidated, there was a shift in the place of birth. This shift needs to be located in the wider context of increasing *medicalization* of pregnancy and childbirth. Medicalization is to identify or categorize a condition or behaviour as being a disorder requiring medical treatment or intervention. A more technological approach to childbirth gained momentum in Europe and North

America throughout the 1700s. Professional male obstetricians were the focus. Over time, female midwives lost status and came to be portrayed as unenlightened and unhygienic. In the 1920s, nearly three-fourths of American births took place at homes. By 1960, 96 per cent took place in hospitals (ibid.). However, by the mid-twentieth century, women perceived childbirth as an impersonal experience. The return to a more natural childbirth was an attempt to defend the meaning in childbirth, which had reduced as pain was removed from the experience. Studies on the effects of drugs on foetal development as well as increasing concern over chemical toxins in the environment resulted in increasing uncertainty regarding the use of anaesthesia in childbirth (ibid.).

From the literature available on the subject, it is clear that in the context of the United States, before the twentieth century, birth was a home affair, where women delivered in the comfort of their familiar surroundings, though infant mortality and maternal mortality was high. Post twentieth century till about the 1950s, birth was a medical event. Urbanization, centralization of health care and improved medical technology brought about better safety for mothers and babies, but increased the social and psychological burden (Norr et al., 1977). Women's role moved from being central to being passive in the birth process while the environment changed from home to hospital. Starting from the 1950s with the Read natural birth (discussed later in the paper) and Lamaze method in the 1960s, in addition to the social movements that pressed for making childbirth a more active experience for women, the situation changed to an extent (ibid.). There was research done subsequently, which proved that excessive medication is harmful for both the mother and the child. However, this would be true only in certain hospitals among the upper-middle-class women. Birth process has a lot of variations and so does women's subjective experiences of birth.

It is not just obstetric or medical factors that have a bearing on the childbirth experience of women, but socio-psychological factors are also important.

> A high status, a close marriage, and less traditional sex role attitudes encourage women to prepare for birth. Preparation encourages greater support from husbands and teaches pain control techniques. The results are greater participation in delivery, less pain, and more enjoyment. (Norr et al., 1977: 270)

OBJECTIVES AND METHODOLOGY

Sociologists and social anthropologists have been interested in understanding the customs, rituals and practices associated with birth. Yet, few researches have asked how women actually perceive and experience childbirth pain or what accounts for their different experiences in the historical and present context.

Childbirth and pain 'management' is a complex subject that has many historical layers to it. It is as much a physiological process as it is a cultural phenomenon. It is not simply about what is best for the mother and child, but it involves a host of sociocultural factors. The objective of the paper is to explore the different facets to this subject and also look at the different debates that surround the issue of pain in childbirth.

The methodology that I have used is review of secondary literature available on this subject in both Indian and Western context to address the objectives of the paper, namely the following:

1. To understand the use of technology in childbirth, its history and its implications;
2. To understand the various phases of childbirth and pain management in the West, starting from twilight sleep to homebirth movement of today; and
3. To understand the situation in India and take into account the differences by caste and class.

THEORETICAL PERSPECTIVE

In this paper, the importance of social and cultural factors is highlighted in the understanding of health in the context of childbirth. As we know, culture plays a very important role in health and illness. It can be argued that the health status of a society is a function of the norms and values of that society. Culture is defined as a system of norms, values and customs that are socially learned by members of a group and are passed from generation to generation. It is the total way of life of people. It derives from societal practices, norms and values, including health habits. The definition of health and health practices of people can only be understood within their cultural context. In addition, time is an important factor as culture is not static, and it changes with time within the same social setting.

Drawing from the above perspective, my paper focuses on the historical trajectory of childbirth in the West, the shift from home to hospital, and in some contexts, back to homebirth today and the sociological analysis of pain and its management through the use of different forms of drugs. The mainstay of this paper is that pain is not a universal and not merely a medical phenomenon that needs treatment, but it needs to be looked at in a sociocultural context since its perception and the way it is handled differ in different cultures.

PAIN MANAGEMENT THROUGH THE USE OF TECHNOLOGY

> Pain is never merely a sensation. It always involves a mental aspect, an idea of its meaning and purpose. It is known that very strong emotional states can change the experience of pain. Labour pain can have negative or positive meaning, depending on whether the child is wanted, the interaction of the labouring woman with those attending her, her sense of ease or disease in the environment provided for birth, her relationship with the father of her child and her attitude to her body throughout the reproductive process. (Kitzinger, 1978: 119)

According to Fox and Worts (1999), it can be said that pain has been a major reason why many women have considered necessary medical assistance during birth. Because of minimal social support in a hospital setting today, many women welcome medical intervention, both out of concern for their babies' welfare and because it promises to leave them in better shape to take up the responsibilities that they would have to fulfil as mothers.

Sedatives tend to prolong labour rather than shorten it in many cases, by diminishing the expulsive forces of the uterine contractions. This adds to the risks for the mother and more so for the child. A proper knowledge of the action of sedative drugs is needed. Although analgesia and anaesthesia may involve risks to the mother and child, most physicians are convinced that an important cause of maternal death rate is less resistance from excessive fatigue and shock (ibid.).

According to Carson (2000), analgesic or sedative drugs are administered in the first and second stages of labour, since pain is relieved without the loss of consciousness in most cases. Anaesthetics are used to make one unconscious, and they are used occasionally in the second stage, whereas deeper anaesthesia is used during delivery. In the nineteenth century, the first analgesics ether and chloroform were used by doctors during birth. In the second decade of the twentieth century, the American National Twilight Sleep Association was formed as a middle- and upper-class feminist organization to demand the use of twilight sleep (ibid.).

As dangers of these drugs were known, women's organizations began to mobilize against these drugs. In the mid-twentieth century, natural childbirth movement began to gain strength and question the meaning of 'painless' birth, viewed pain as a natural part of childbirth and believed that they can be managed through breathing techniques and psychological orientations rather than drugs (Hollen, 2003). Despite this, the use of anaesthesia, particularly epidurals that suppress the experience of pain without changing woman's consciousness, is on the rise today (ibid.).

THE TWILIGHT SLEEP MOVEMENT

If we need to understand women's reaction to the isolation and lack of control that have characterized twentieth-century childbirth, it is necessary to focus on the twilight sleep movement in America, which involves the use of the scopolamine and morphine that removed memories of labour from women's minds. In this, the women went to sleep and delivered their babies. The drug altered their consciousness so that they did not remember painful labours, and their bodies did not feel fatigued by their efforts. Both the women who demanded scopolamine and the doctors who agreed to use it saw it as far superior to other anaesthesia because it did not restrain muscle function and could be administered throughout the birthing process (Leavitt, 1980).

From a present-day feminist perspective, as Leavitt points out, the use of such drugs would clearly indicate women's passivity in the birth process. But in 1914–15, at the height of the twilight sleep movement, many women viewed the painless childbirth as a right. She argues that for twilight sleep advocates, loss of control during the sleep was less important than their determination to control the decision about what kind of labour they would want (ibid.).

Paradoxically, by encouraging women to sleep during their deliveries, the twilight sleep movement detached women from their bodies. In this condition, most women from the 1920s to the 1960s did not experience one of their bodies' powerful actions (ibid.). The twilight sleep movement helped change the definition of birthing from a natural home event, as it was in the nineteenth century, to an illness requiring hospitalization.

> Parturient feminists today, seeking fully to experience childbirth, paradoxically need to fight a tradition of drugged, hospital-controlled births, itself the partial result of their own past struggle to increase women's control over their bodies. (Leavitt, 1980: 156)

However, there were many cases where the drugs were not administered correctly since it required special care, expertise and resources of the hospital. Leavitt has also quoted doctors saying to popular magazines and newspapers on the need for such a drug for middle- and upper-class women who were less enduring to pain as opposed to women from lower classes that perform more physical labour and can withstand more pain.

TRANSFORMATION FROM 'TWILIGHT SLEEP' TO NATURAL CHILDBIRTH

According to Fox and Worts (1999), the American perceptions of birth transformed from the twilight sleep in 1914 to the emergence of the natural childbirth movement in the 1940s and 1950s. The shift is seen as a result of the reduction in maternal mortality that took place between 1937 and 1945 and also the publication of 'Childbirth Without Fear' in 1943 by the British obstetrician Grantly Dick-Read. Those two factors played a prominent role in bringing in a new era of natural childbirth with a well-judged use of drugs and importance given to personal satisfaction of the women.

Pain, according to Dr Read, is the result of fear that causes tension in the cervix at the time when the longitudinal muscles of the uterus are at work to dilate the cervix. The resulting muscle disharmony is the cause of pain in labour. If fear could be overcome, he said, tension in the cervix would decrease and labour would require strength but relatively be painless (ibid.).

Proponents of the Read method deals with the pregnant mother's tensions by correcting false information, explaining her the facts of normal labour and delivery, and educating her to relax and accept childbirth as a happy experience. A technique of slow, abdominal breathing learned in childbirth classes assists the mother (Ulin, 1963).

The *Lamaze method* has its roots in the Pavlovian conditioned response theory. It is a technique of very rapid, shallow respiration with great intensity and concentration. The woman learns that this respiratory response must come at the first sign of each contraction and last till the contraction ends. The unprepared woman's natural reaction to a painful contraction is either restlessness or panic. As a result, the pain increases. The prepared woman, however, is able to inhibit the pain by substituting this self-controlled respiratory activity to her contractions (ibid.).

INCREASING USE OF TECHNOLOGY IN CHILDBIRTH

Caesarean Section

According to Selin and Stone (2009), prior to the nineteenth century, caesarean section was used only in rare cases and mortality associated with it was very high, as high as 80–90 per cent in the eighteenth century, which gradually lowered towards the twentieth century but still remained high when compared to women giving birth vaginally. In the 1990s and early 2000s, the overall rates of caesarean delivery have been at high levels; in 2008, this figure rose to 30 births out of 100 in the United States.

As pregnancy and birth stress women biologically, the addition of surgery results in higher rates of infection, haemorrhage and even death. Scholars argue that modern medicine views birth process through a very narrow lens because of which Western medicine supports caesarean delivery as an appropriate tool in managed birth care. This acceptance and use of caesarean section is often *not* directed by biological need but by product of American medical model of birth (ibid.).

The rates of anaesthesia use in obstetrics have gone up rapidly on an international level in recent years, generally in response to consumer demand (Carson, 2000). Anxiety often accompanies the prolonged pain that many women experience during childbirth. For nearly all of the women interviewed by Fox and Worts in one of their studies, anxiety was a major component of the experience of giving birth for the first time. However, the medical intervention aimed at reducing pain often served to enhance women's fears. For many of the women interviewed, medical procedures added to worries about their own and their babies' well-being. Several women described becoming frightened at the prospect of medical procedures, especially caesarean section. The use of medical technology undermined many women's confidence and, as a result, often generated a desire for more intervention (Fox and Worts, 1999). Thus, it can be argued that medical intervention promises pain relief, yet it may come at the cost of increased anxiety for the woman.

Episiotomy

Episiotomy is a surgical procedure for widening the outlet of the birth canal to facilitate delivery of the baby. It is now a common practice in obstetrics across countries. It is a routine procedure in most deliveries, even the so-called natural birth. Perhaps most women do not even know if they can ask their doctors not to perform an episiotomy and they suffer from episiotomy pain during the first week of post-partum.

Epidural Analgesia

According to Madorossian (2003), in the West, medicalization of birth is taking place at the same time as hospitals are adopting rhetoric of 'natural' childbirth and family-centred maternity care. Medical institutions across the country are now sponsoring childbirth classes that are based on alternative models of childbirth (the Lamaze and Read methods) and encourage couples to become participants in 'natural' childbirth. Despite the time, resources and energy that are spent representing it as the ideal form of delivery, most couples enter the labour room determined to have a natural childbirth and leave it after having an epidural analgesia to obtain pain relief without the loss of consciousness. Couples do not realize the minimal effect on pain these natural childbirth techniques are likely to have in a hospital setting since such techniques are not designed for high-tech hospitals that place time limits on labour and seek to speed up contractions (ibid.).

Since hospitals encourage natural childbirth and a high percentage of couples give up on it during labour, author questions why the mainstream is not holding these institutions responsible for this high rate of failure. Instead of giving up trying to have a natural childbirth in the hospital, expectant mothers are increasingly giving up on natural childbirth itself (ibid.).

THE INDIAN CONTEXT

Homebirth in India today is either in existence in rural areas or amongst some sections of the urban poor. It is because middle- and upper-class women in urban areas have little or no access to lay midwives or nurse midwives in hospital that they can approach independent of the doctors as is the case in the United States or Germany (Naraindas et al., forthcoming). For most urban educated women, homebirth is seen as 'risky'. The Indian state promotes institutional birthing as the solution to the high rate of infant and maternal mortality. Despite this, according to NFHS statistics, in 1992–93 the rate of infant mortality at home and in the hospital was exactly the same for rural India; in urban India, it was 34.1 deaths per thousand at home as against 31.3 in public health facilities (ibid.).

Institutional delivery has become so popular that while the WHO gives the directive of 10 per cent rate for episiotomies, it is almost 100 per cent in private hospitals and 98 per cent in tertiary government hospitals. While caesareans vary between 7 per cent and 25 per cent in the Europe and America, it is close to 45 per cent or more in private hospitals in a city like Chennai (ibid.). In India, a caesarean section is seen not only as 'painless', but it is also seen as a sign of status and modernity, whereas homebirth is seen as backward and risky. There is a discussion possible around a birth by operation, but there is usually a 'silence' around the vaginal birth, as it is often seen as a matter of shame and ritual pollution (ibid.).

MANAGEMENT OF CHILDBIRTH PAIN IN TAMIL NADU

In a study of rural women in Kanathur-Reddikuppam district of Tamil Nadu, Cecilia Van Hollen conducted fieldwork and interviewed many women, doctors, healthcare workers and found several interesting similarities and differences between women in the West and in Tamil Nadu in their use of technology to manage pain. While Robbie Davis Floyd points to an increase in the use of analgesics among American women, the women in Tamil Nadu were using oxytocin to increase labour, but were not even aware of anaesthesia as an option. While the American women fear the prospect of using pitocin without anaesthesia to induce their labour, women in Tamil Nadu were just demanding to be induced without the idea of anaesthesia (Hollen, 2003).

Vali means pain or ache in Tamil and *piracava vali* refers to both the pain and the function the pain serves, that is, contractions, no distinction is made between the two in the language (ibid.). That is why women here believe that childbirth is not possible without pain (which also means contractions). *Vali* also means strength or power, therefore it is the combination of pain and danger that women must endure during childbirth and it is in this context that women in Tamil culture are constructed as fearless beings (ibid.). Due to the effects of modernity, women wanted to be induced because they could no longer withstand the long, drawn-out pain of labour, and they got induced with oxytocin shots to get over the pain quickly. They also believed that a quick labour would be safer for the baby as the time taken would be less (ibid.).

Some older women in this study said that not only had women's tolerance of pain lessened these days, but their bodies had also changed as they were no longer getting the contractions that they got in the past, hence the need to induce labour (ibid.). Another reason why these women readily accepted medicines to induce labour is that they already have a tradition of making herbal medicines at home which serve the same purpose. These are known as *kasayams* (herbal homemade medicines). There were many *kasayams* to induce labour, but no *kasayam* to reduce pain. Common ingredients are ginger, jiggery, cumin and coriander. However, these were not seen as substitutes for oxytocin. *Kasayam* confirmed whether labour had begun and oxytocin confirmed that it would be over quickly (ibid.).

Apart from these, there were also politicoeconomic constraints that led to use of oxytocin. One of them is crowd control. Since government hospitals could not accommodate the huge crowd, they often had to fasten labour to move women from prenatal to delivery ward as quickly as possible so as to accommodate more women (ibid.).

In many homebirths also, oxytocin drugs would be used as injections or drips with glucose purchased from local pharmacists. Often, the local health care workers would do so in homebirths where the women would now have both access to oxytocin and emotional support at home (Jeffery and Jeffery, 2009).

Studies in several parts of South Asia indicate that oxytocin is already readily available outside the formal health care system, even in remote rural areas. In rural home deliveries, when oxytocin is arranged, it is used to increase rather than induce labour (ibid.). Most reports say that it is administered not by intravenous infusion but by intramuscular injection, which means that the effective dose cannot be measured or regulated. Usually, it is administered by local rural practitioners, with or without training. Such use can result in undesirable outcomes, including uterine rupture and foetal asphyxia (ibid.).

Many sources have suggested that the needle is a powerful sign of 'modernity' since the intra-partum injections were more common among women of higher socio-economic status and among relatively more educated women, suggesting that oxytocin was used less because of need and more because of the ability to pay, and is associated with 'modernity' (ibid.).

DIFFERENCES BY RACE, ETHNICITY AND CLASS

It has been frequently stated that modes of expression of pain differ among different cultures and within cultural groups (Winsberg and Greenlick, 1967). There is variation in how births are managed based on race, ethnicity and class. For instance, the same technological intervention may be interpreted and experienced in different ways by different women in the United States (Hollen, 2003). Some argue that women in higher socio-economic brackets experience greater degrees of technological intervention, whereas some others argue the opposite. Patients with Medicaid in the United States are sometimes not provided with epidurals, unless they pay for it themselves due to higher cost of administering it.

In 'childbirth without pain in Italy', it has been argued how the head of council of the Roman Catholic Church in Italy wrote in a book on morality that a woman who suffers the pain of childbirth without use of anaesthesia is a more Christian mother, although there is no harm if a woman opts for it owing to fear of the pain (Wilcox, 1967).

In the same book, the following lines can be found under the section titled 'pregnancy':

> Anaesthesia of the woman in labor is not forbidden, provided that it is done in such a way as to bring no damage to the mother or to the product of conception. It can be recommended to those women who, fearing the pains of childbirth, are opposed to becoming pregnant.

It is further argued that psychological and social factors play an important role among those who rejected anaesthesia in Italian hospital of those times. Traditional mentality, the attitudes of the woman's husband and family, the influence of the Church's former teachings, created in the pregnant woman the idea that childbirth should occur without intervention except in extreme cases, and that to permit intervention is disgraceful. The increasing numbers of women who had heard of the means to prevent suffering were psychologically caught between the wish to avoid pain and the inhibitions imposed by this taboo (ibid.).

In Tamil Nadu also there were certain differences in practice when it came to the use of analgesics. The women here who were aware of the use of such drugs for reducing pain felt that these were meant for upper- and middle-class women who could not tolerate the pain and needed anaesthesia. Hence, these were more frequently used in private rather than government hospitals (Hollen, 2003).

RETURN TO HOMEBIRTH MOVEMENT

As I have discussed earlier, while post 1920s, caesareans, epidurals and heavy doses of pain medication became the norm, in the 1960s and 1970s; women began to question and challenge the way obstetricians were treating them as if childbirth were a disease. Women began to make efforts to regain their power, and the homebirth movement was born in the United States.

Today, there is a resurgence of people wanting to make all of pregnancy and birth a family experience in countries such as the United States and Germany. The homebirth movement there is an alternative health belief system that promotes a model of childbirth different from the biomedical model. This stresses non-intervention and it promotes individual responsibility for health care. Members of this movement are typically highly educated, upper-class, white women.

According to Mardorossian (2003), a carefully supervised homebirth in combination with good nutrition and care has been proven to be very safe for women. Today, the ones who believe in homebirths, especially in the United States, are committed and have faith in their body's natural ability to give birth. They devote time and energy to find the right birth practitioner after doing a research. Homebirth practitioners include naturopaths, family practitioners, nurses, physician's assistants, chiropractors and midwives.

Therefore, while in the United States and Germany, the natural birth movement resulted in a section of upper-class white women to prefer consulting a nurse midwife rather than doctor and to give birth naturally, that is, without a caesarean, episiotomy or even epidural, in India this is not the case. Here, one would find few urban educated, upper-class women in private hospitals who have not had a caesarean section. It is believed that a caesarean is either painless or that women are ready to exchange the pain of surgery for the pain of labour (Naraindas et al., forthcoming).

CONCLUSION

Medical practice is always developed in the context of changing cultural and social values. The biomedical model of birth emerged with the Industrial Revolution, which completely took over childbirth and advocated that hospital birth with certain technological interventions is the safest for the mother and child. It gradually dismissed natural births attended by family and midwives as 'risky'. It assumed that maternal and child mortality can be lowered by the use of technology.

A labouring woman even in popular media is depicted as trying to rush to the hospital and screaming for pain medication and is never portrayed as being calm and in control. Pain is depicted as being excruciating and in need of management through anaesthesia. Medical anthropologists have shown that pain itself has some social significance in many cultures that has been changed by the use of anaesthesia. The return to a more natural childbirth in the 1950s and 1960s and its revival today can be seen as an effort to preserve the meaning in childbirth. As per the feminist debate, it is seen as one in which women want to regain control over the birthing process and want to do away with male-dominated birth management. Some see medicalization as controlling and others see it as liberating since women today have a choice as to the kind of birth they want to have and can demand for pain relief that was inconceivable a few decades back.

However, the picture is not so simple. The question is whether women actually have control over medical procedures once they are admitted as 'patients' in the hospitals. As part of another research that is ongoing, I have interviewed several women who had wanted normal delivery but ended up having caesarean without a clear understanding of what went 'wrong'. Even episiotomy and epidural has become routine procedures in the so-called natural delivery. There are also differences by ethnicity and class since what women want ranges from simple care in the hospital to control over birth process, depending on their access to knowledge and resources (Lazarus, 1994).

There was a time when upper- and middle-class women sought pain relief and associated it with modernity, and today it is again such women who want to embrace pain and experience childbirth. As discussed earlier, on the one hand, rural women in Tamil Nadu want to experience pain as pain and contractions are inseparable concepts in their culture and, on the other hand, educated and high-class women in the United States today also want to experience pain through natural homebirth. A lot of people today question the validity of modern medicine in the context of childbirth and that could be the reason why modern hospitals encourage natural childbirth, give coaching classes that teach appropriate breathing techniques so that women who want to experience natural childbirth do so in the hospital itself and need not go to midwives.

REFERENCES

Carson, Carolyn Leonard, 2000, '*Review: What a Blessing She Had Chloroform: The Medical and Social Response to the Pain of Childbirth from 1800 to the Present*. By Donald Caton. New Haven: Yale University Press', *Journal of Social History*, 34(2): 469–71.

Dye, Schrom Nancy, 1980, 'History of Childbirth in America', *Women: Sex and Sexuality*, 6(1): 97–108.

Fox, Bonnie and Diana Worts, 1999, 'Revisiting the Critique of Medicalized Childbirth: A Contribution to the Sociology of Birth', *Gender and Society*, 13(3): 326–46.

Hollen, Van Cecilia, 2003, *Birth on the Threshold: Childbirth and Modernity in South India*. California: University of California Press.

Jeffery, Roger and Patricia Jeffery, 2009, *Labour Management: Oxytocin in the Context of the Millennium Development Goals in Tracing Pharmaceuticals in South Asia*. Edinburgh: University of Edinburgh.

Kitzinger, Sheila, 1978, 'Pain in Childbirth', *Journal of Medical Ethics*, 4(3): 119–121.

Lazarus, Ellen, 1994, 'What Do Women Want: Issues of Choice, Control, and Class in Pregnancy and Childbirth', *Medical Anthropology Quarterly*, 8(1): 25–46.

Leavitt, Walzer Judith, 1980, 'Birthing and Anaesthesia: The Debate over Twilight Sleep', *Women: Sex and Sexuality*, 6(1): 147–64.

Mardorossian, Carine M., 2003, 'Labouring Women, Coaching Men: Masculinity and Childbirth Education in the Contemporary United States', *Hypatia*, 18(3): 113–34.

Naraindas, H., J. Quack and W. Sax, forthcoming, *Asymmetrical Conversations: Contestations, Circumventions and Blurring of Therapeutic Boundaries*.

Norr, L. Kathleen, Carolyn R. Block, Allan Charles, Suzanne Meyering and Ellen Meyers, 1977, 'Explaining Pain and Enjoyment in Childbirth', *Journal of Health and Social Behaviour*, 18(3): 260–75.

Selin, Helaine and Pamela Stone, 2009, *Childbirth across Cultures: Ideas and Practices of Pregnancy, Childbirth and Postpartum*. Netherlands: Springer Publications.

Ulin, Richardson Priscilla, 1963, 'The Exhilarating Moment of Birth', *The American Journal of Nursing*, 63(6): 60–7.

Wilcox, M. Isobel, 1967, 'Childbirth without Pain in Italy', *The Journal of Sex Research*, 3(2): 180–81.

Winsberg, B. and M. Greenlick, 1967, 'Pain Response in Negro and White Obstetrical Patients', *Journal of Health and Social Behaviour*, 8(3): 222–27.

CHAPTER 7

Reproductive Repertoire: Making Sense of Common Sense

Mohd. Shahid

The reproductive patterns of Indian women are commonly painted as tales of pregnancy and childbirth, which are too early, too soon, too many and too late. There is a widespread assumption that 'people in rural India go on producing children as long as they can' (Enke, 1966; Endres, 1975), and on the same token, it is also argued that 'the early marriage provides a longer duration of procreation resulting in more childbirths and vice-versa' (Wyron and Gordon, 1971; Mandelbaum, 1974). However, Patel (2006) countered these arguments and observed that even social onomastics reinforces ideas about desirability or otherwise of childbirth during certain stages in a couple's fertility trajectory. Patel's study further showed that

> couples know the permissible range within which their fertility behaviour can vary. They know when the number of children is less or more than required, and what their optimum number and sex composition should be. Even the young unmarried children know the fertility norms and react with surprise if other's fertility performance falls short of the customary expectations. (ibid.: 86–7)

It would be interesting to see how social and cultural factors govern and contribute in developing the normative discourse on marriage and fertility. How do people make sense of the marriage and fertility issues, and to what extent socio-cultural context guides and governs the popular perception? Is the popular *common sense* on issues of marriage and fertility, in general, and pregnancy and childbirth, in particular, hegemonic in nature? Does it represent dominant constructions and legitimize biasness and prejudices for the *other*—they may be women (gender-based discrimination), rural population (region-specific stereotypes), minorities (religion-centric prejudices) and many more such groups on the other side of the power spectrum? This paper focuses on some such questions and endeavours to interrogate how popular common sense upholds and sustains the hegemonic constructions on the issues of marriage and fertility and how this popular common sense on marriage and fertility also discriminates across gender, region and religion. A twofold approach is adopted for conceptualization and discussion. First, to collate and put to discussion major narratives on marriage and fertility deriving from secondary data as also from the authors' own personal experiences of growing up in Uttar Pradesh, coupled with research experiences in western Uttar Pradesh. Second, it strives to reinterpret the collated reproductive narratives with the Gramscian notion of common sense.

REPRODUCTIVE REPERTOIRE AND *COMMON SENSE*

There is a no better way to gain an understanding of a society than through its stock of stories, which constitute its dramatic resources (Kakar, 1990: 3). It is rightly noted that 'since the ultimate reality can only be apprehended experientially, its hue, flavour and ramifications for ordinary life are best conveyed to the uninitiated mass of people in the culture through story-myth, fable, parable, and the tale-thus further elevating the prestige of the narrative form' (ibid.). Every child in India is exposed to stock narratives across a plethora of issues, and marriage and fertility are no exceptions. Marriage, pregnancy and childbirth constitute important markers of *rites of passage* across societies. In India, there are culturally approved notions, rites and rituals denoting prescriptions and proscriptions, celebration or no celebration on the events relating to marriage and fertility in general, and pregnancy and childbirth, in particular. These constitute collective memory, and narratives around these may vary across cultures, but in each culture these are passed on from generation to generation. It is this inventory of narratives and markers on the issues of fertility, marriage, pregnancy and childbirth that we have referred as the reproductive repertoire. It takes the form of popular common sense.

Gramsci has a distinct meaning and understanding for the common sense derived mainly from his Italian notion metamorphosed with his political Marxist philosophy. 'Unlike English, the Italian notion of common sense (*senso commune*) does not so much mean good, sound, practical sense rather it means normal or average understanding. So in Italian, a good sense (*buon senso*) is more distinct from common sense than in English' (Ives, 2004: 74). Forgacs (2000: 421) defines the Gramscian common sense: 'Everyone has a number of *conceptions of the world*, ... Many of these conceptions are imposed and absorbed passively from outside, or from the past, and are accepted and lived uncritically. In this case, they constitute what Gramsci calls common sense.' Many elements in popular common sense contribute to people's subordination by making situations of inequality and oppression appear to them as natural and unchangeable (ibid.). It is in this way that we attempt to understand how the popular common sense around reproductive repertoire discriminates across gender, region and religion and how it legitimizes the biases and stereotypes.

MARRIAGE—THE SACRED DUTY; FIRST CHILD—THE TEST OF FERTILITY

Theoretically, marriage is seen as a sacrament and a contract in Hinduism and Islam, respectively. But irrespective of the religious groups, the popular common sense places marriage as a significantly important responsibility. Popular common sense also puts the onus more on the parents than on the prospective marrying persons. It is considered an important duty of parents and is a marker of responsible parentage. The marrying off of all the children is considered an achievement of proud parents who have performed their last important responsibility. And probably, it also speaks of early marriages or low age at marriage. Looking through the gender prism, however, one finds that it is the marriage of daughters that attracts more attention. The onset of puberty sets the grounds for the parents' unreasonably high concern for the marriage of their daughters. In consequence, females become the victims of early marriage and of the collateral damages of curtailment of education, career and dignified living. Thus, the popular common sense governing the sacred duty of marriage covers the way in which women are conveniently placed in the vicious circle of life-long disempowerment.

Unlike marriage (rather early marriage of daughters), which is singularly the priority agenda of parents, the issue of childbirth becomes the top-priority agenda for both the newly married couples and their parents as also of the significant others. It is observed that the average age of women at first childbirth has shown an increasing trend during 1972–91 in all the major states, but this change has been very nominal (Pathak and Singh, 1995: 184). Patel (2006: 58), in her Rajasthan study, found that nearly 55 per cent of women became mothers before crossing the age of 20 years, 28 per cent between the ages of 21 and 25 years and over 4 per cent after 25 years of age. The National Family Health Survey-III (NFHS-3) has provided that the percentage of women marrying before 18 years has come down to 45 per cent (NFHS-3) from 50 per cent in NFHS-2 and the median age at first childbirth is 19.8 years (IIPS, 2007).

Studying human fertility in India, Mandelbaum (1974) observed that 'for a young wife, pregnancy is fine, the baby is fun, motherhood is grand and God given.' We are recalled of the anguish of a young woman aged 20 years who did not experience a pregnancy even after two years of married life. She was highly disturbed on not bearing a child/pregnancy even after two years of her marriage. She shared that now she had started encountering a series of questions/whispers/stories as to why she had not experienced childbirth even after two 'long' years of marriage? The first pregnancy/childbirth is a test of one's fertility, which is expected from women/newly wed daughters-in-law, she also wants to pass it at the earliest. Patel (2006) noted that motherhood is extolled, whereas barrenness is held as a curse. The popular common sense provides space not only for the celebration of the first childbirth, but there are notable prescriptions, rites and rituals for the declaration of the very first pregnancy. And the young woman becomes the centre for all these celebrations and felicitations. A hero is made of her for fulfilling the expectations and desires of the family. But just as pregnancy and childbirth are extolled, barrenness is bitterly cursed. The brunt of this barrenness falls on the woman. She is questioned for the delay in childbirth. She is made solely responsible for the barrenness. The popular common sense relates and interprets the fertility of earth and the fertility of women. Despite the progress in medical sciences and scientific tests proving that either partner, irrespective of male (husband) or female (wife), could be responsible for childbirth; the woman bears the onus of responsibility for the misfortune. Innumerable number of cases have come up in which women are maltreated, deserted and divorced because they failed to pass the 'test of fertility' for which as per popular common sense, they are solely responsible. We have come across real-life cases during field studies, as also the tales in the process of growing up in Indian society, whereby the polygamous marriages, especially the practice of bigamy, is overtly justified on the grounds that there have been no childbirths in the first marriage, how long should one wait! And in cases where there were no children from second marriage as well, then too people especially the old women lamented on the poor fellow's destiny instead of exploring the cause of infertility in men. Probably, in popular common sense men were always virile and virile men could not be infertile! This is how popular common sense has contributed to obscure the reality, cover the discrimination and legitimize oppression. Many a times, the marginalized sections themselves became the flag bearers of their own oppression. It is observed that in most instances of infertility or delayed childbirth, it is the old ladies especially the mothers-in-law who are most concerned, and it is they who coax the young husbands to look for alternatives in the form of separation, desertion, divorce or polygamy for the want of child. This exhibits how hegemony works, not so much by coercion but with the force of consent and by making people do things at odds with their own interest (Gramsci, 1971).

Baby Boy: The Divine Reward

'May you be the mother of a hundred sons?' This is the metaphorical wish young brides generously receive in India across religions and regions, with variations only in framing of the text than in actual substance – the wish for son birth(s). *Doodoh nahao puto falo* (May there be showering of wealth and son births) is the popular tale and the wish we kept hearing. The louder message is that the birth of male child is the divine reward. Bumiller (1991) travelling over the length and breadth of the country, interacting and interviewing women, was so moved that she titled her travelogue *May You Be the Mother of a Hundred Sons: A Journey Among the Women of India. Patel* (2006: 87) was amazed when during her fieldwork in a Rajasthan village, 13-year-old Buddha reminded her that one son is no son just as one eye is no eye (*ek ankh main ankh nahin ne ek put main put nee*). Almost similarly, an old lady clarified the calculus of at least two sons to Ashish Bose (1988) during his field visits to Rajasthan in the 1980s. We still have the refreshing memory of a casual discussion with a staff member in a Central University who in the process of explaining the gentleness and increasing prosperity of one of his relatives suddenly paused and said they (the relative couple) have only two daughters and then again paused and said they must have indulged in some sin and that is why they do not have a son. God rewards and the greatest reward of all is the blessing of a son.

Popular common sense has a *karma* theory to son birth. Among Hindus, privileged are the parents who have sons, for sons will further pave the way for *Moksha* (salvation). Although Muslims consider the birth of a daughter a mark of *Sunnat* (saying and practice of Prophet Mohammad), but the differential celebrations that mark the birth of a son compared with a daughter speak volumes about the *baby boy, divine reward* thesis. Even the naming of children and the order of male childbirth many a times explains the rationale of the total number of childbirths the couple have had. The name *Pancham* or *Pachchu* explains that the boy must be born as the fifth child after the four female births. Unusual equations of male–female children, say five females and one male child, clearly indicate that females have been born in the quest for a male child. Bose (1995: 8) has coined the term *demographic fundamentalism*, that is, the craze for sons and the relentless efforts to try and get a son even when five or six daughters have been born. Basu (1994) has also argued that every observer or resident within the Indian scene has personal knowledge of at least a handful of homes where childbearing has continued mercilessly until a son has been born even when this has meant a string of five, six or even seven and more daughters first. Tragically, in the popular common sense, such episodes of demographic fundamentalism are not condemned or cornered, instead the community feels satisfied that finally a son is being gifted to the family. This is how patriarchy has coloured the common perception that fails to perceive the decolouring of the world of women.

Chimera of the Two Child Norm

'Ham do, Hamare do' (We Two, Ours Two) was and still is the popular slogan of India's family welfare programme popularizing the two-child norm. It was also promoted as a great value symbolizing nationalism. The increasing population of India was considered a grave threat to the nation and national interest, and hence birth control and limiting the family size to the two-child norm was a significant step forward for the cause of the nation. The banners, billboards, hoardings, buses

and walls all started propagating this two-child norm. Government machinery, as also the international donor agencies in unison, was on the mission mode to place the notion of the two-child norm on the pedestal of common wisdom. In consequence, the parents with only two children were acknowledged as enlightened couples with a vision for the nation. The urban educated elite emerged as the champions of nationalism and the two-child norm. Resultantly, popular common sense painted the poor, uneducated and rural as a category of people who were not in a position to understand the issues of national interest and hence failing to adhere to the two-child norm. Another category of perpetual defaulters in the popular parlance were the Muslims, who were projected as constituencies never cared for national interest and who had a natural propensity to profligate.

The figures of Census 2001, NFHS-3 (2005–06), and Census 2011 have exposed the brutal realities under the cover of the two-child norm. The abnormally declining juvenile sex ratio amply illustrated in Census 2001 and 2011 confirms the thesis of son preference and the brutal elimination of girls even before birth. More alarming is the fact that the number of such DEMARU (Daughter [Elimination] Maru) states has increased from Census 2001 to Census 2011 (Bose, 2006; Census, 2011). The analysis of the results of the NFHS-3 has demystified the notion of rural, illiterate population and disempowered mothers contributing or remaining moot spectator to female infanticide. NFHS-3 figures have highlighted that female sex-selective abortions are more concentrated in urban metropolitan and in the population cohort, which is in general educated and economically sound, and wherein women, in particular, are educationally and economically empowered. Why so? What does this imply? The only answer seems to be that preference for son is part and parcel of common wisdom. Patriarchy has infiltrated and colonized our cognitive frame. Despite higher educational qualifications, economic prosperity and women autonomy (in terms of education, income and mobility), we have failed to challenge patriarchy, and hence the perpetuation of preference for son continues unabatedly.

A very important phenomenon that is noted is that the urban, educated, economically well off and the champions of two child norm have adopted and promoted this norm as a value in national interest, but paradoxically practise it with a calculus of at least one son. This has probably become the major cause for the increasing percentage of sex-selective abortions. It is told and recorded in studies as well that the birth of the first child used to be left on chance. Patel (2006) noted that in the instance of first childbirth, people first ask for the health of mother and child and then about the sex of child. However, in many of recent discussions, we are told that now the couple wants to ensure a son in the very first pregnancy. If this is coming up as popular common sense, then the future is certainly bleak. It is here that those advocating the small family norm, which is a fine proposition, should have to understand and accept that popular common sense had given the cover to urban, educated and elite sections of society to promote the two-child norm with a skewed sex ratio.

The penchant for the two-child norm, the issue of nationalism and the Rightwing advocacy for non-demographic objectives have been unfortunately successful in developing the common perception that Muslims profligate and are majorly responsible for the increasing population. The popular common perception is more strengthened by the mischievous interpretation of national-level figures and depicting that Muslim fertility is higher than the other religious groups. At this juncture, suffice is to mention that there is a great North–South divide in terms of achieving the replenishment-level population growth rate. Many of the southern states have even moved towards negative growth rate of population. But many of the Northern states are far behind the replenishment-level population growth rate (Bose, 2006). The majority of Muslim population is concentrated in states with a high growth rate of population and in those states Muslims' fertility rate resembles that of majority of the religious groups. Hence, there is a need to have a disaggregated analysis of data and understand the layers of disparities rather than concealing these to present the negative image of Muslims.

Welcome to the Daughters' Club

Thankfully, we are also encountering the motion to welcome daughters. In many of the formal and informal forums, one has noticed the murmur *welcome to the daughters' club*. Many parents who moved to adhere to the two-child norm and had two daughters were found to be highly contended and satisfied. But to their dissatisfaction, they kept on encountering an innumerable number of queries on *why only two daughters*. Many of the so-called great well-wishers tend to suggest to these parents to move further and have at least one son even if it means few more children or sex-selective abortion. Gramsci

(1971) noted that language can be hegemonizing, but it can also be an instrument of liberation. The notions such as *daughters' club* need to be promoted to occupy the space of popular common sense and works as an anti-hegemony strategy to make dent into patriarchy and fanatic quest for son birth.

Saffron Demography: *Hum Do Hamare Do; Woh Paanch Unke Pachees*

'Saffron demography' rests on claims that there are essential differences between Hindu and Muslim population dynamics in India. The central tenets comprise a set of pernicious myths that have been repeated so often, and with so much authority by Right-wing Hindu politicians, that they have become part of a 'common wisdom' (Jeffery and Jeffery, 2006: 1). The book *Hindus: A Dying Race* published in 1909 by U.N. Mukherji still serves the purpose of those thriving on sectarian politics, and it helps creating an illusion of destiny that Muslims would surpass the Hindu population and the Hindu nation. Deeply riddled with inaccuracies in making predictions about the future and based on absolutely no rational thesis, the book nevertheless provided 'demographic common sense functioning as a trope for extinction' (Datta, 1999: 23 cited in Rao, 2004: 264). The slogan '*Hum do hamare do; Woh panch unke pachees,*' has been frequently used, to borrow from Amartya Sen (2006), to create an illusion of destiny (Muslims overtaking Hindus) and fermenting violence. For example, politico-religious leader Sadhavi Ritambhara used it in her inflammatory speeches (Basu, 1997: 9). The slogan also won the leader of the genocide in Gujarat in 2002 such a shameful but resounding electoral victory (Rao, 2004: 263).

The Hindu Right rhetoric then rests on crucial but false assumptions that polygamy is common among Muslims but unknown among Hindus and that it is associated with high fertility; that Muslim population will soon swamp the Hindu majority in absolute numbers; that Islam is opposed to family planning (Basu, 1997: 9; Jeffery and Jeffery, 2006: 31). Jeffery and Jeffery (2006) on the basis of their decades of ethnographic study in Bijnore, Uttar Pradesh, noted that despite the Hindu Right's complaints about Muslim polygamous marriages (and the censorious comments of many high-caste Hindus in Bijnore about Muslims and polygamy), the proportion of Muslim men with more than one wife remained very small.

Unfortunately, popular common sense on the above issues speaks volumes about the success of the pernicious propaganda of the Right wing. Interestingly, the Muslims' response or the popular common sense supplements the Right-wing assertions. The Right-wing proclaims that Muslims have polygamous marriages and any Muslim child would proudly say four wives are permitted in Islam. The Right-wing states that Muslims have high fertility and Islam opposes family planning; Muslims would encounter that Almighty Allah will take care of the children! Is the actual reality similar to what is proposed?

If not, why are Muslims simply supplementing the Right-wing assertions? Are they conscious of it? Why are they taking a position contradictory to their own interest? Gramsci helps answer these. Unlike the Marxian notion of false consciousness, Gramsci (1971) advocated the notion of contradictory consciousness, which is based on half truth and half falsehood. How is it used determines whether it is used for sustaining hegemony or promoting counter-hegemony. Let us have a quick and close look at this. It was only in the 1971 Census that a report on polygynous marriages in India was published, which provided that polygyny was higher among the *Adivasis* (15.25 per cent) followed by Buddhists (7.9 per cent), Jains (6.72 per cent), Hindus (5.80 per cent) and Muslims (5.70 per cent) (GOI, 1975 cited in Shariff and Razzack, 2006: 104). It is said that in order to avoid sectarian conflicts and adhere to the doctrine of secularism, the religion-wise details were not given. Instead, in reality, the non-availability of actual facts and figures across religious categories became the cause for mythical construction and fermenting pernicious and malicious propaganda against the Muslims. It may also be noted that some Arab countries such as Tunisia have abolished polygyny on the grounds that although the Koranic *sura* permits taking up to four wives, the condition upon which it is based can never be fulfilled. It is impossible to be fair among wives. It negates the possibility of polygyny (Obermeyer, 1994: 45). On the issues of family planning, the Koran neither prescribes nor proscribes it; there is no mention of family planning, but the holy text does command proper care and protection of children. Many of the Muslim countries have launched official family planning programmes. In India, the overall modern contraceptive prevalence rate is 48.5 per cent (37.3 per cent female sterilization, 5.3 per cent condoms, 3.1 per cent pills, 1.8 per cent IUDs and 1 per cent male sterilization) (IIPS,

2007). Our research experiences in rural and urban areas of Aligarh have shown that there is a high prevalence of traditional contraceptive concoctions, among the Hindu and Muslim women. It is being documented that a good number of traditional concoctions are in currency and are used differently (hot or cold or powder form) for abortion as also to avoid conception and starting the menstruation cycle. Despite the fact that women do have stories of how their fellow neighbours died because of the ill effects of traditional contraceptive concoctions, they still prescribe to it. *This probably reflects the poor awareness and availability of modern contraceptives*. And probability gets conformity when you hear their desperate needs for sterilization as also for spacing methods especially among the younger ones. But the discussion with women from both the religious groups illustrates how they see sterilization and how it is an issue of human rights for them. In their common understanding, sterilization is considered equivalent to getting barren, which is abhorred in both the religious groups. In the Indian cultural context, fertility is extolled but barrenness is cursed. There is a notion in both the religious groups that sterilization is not ethical, and there are also tales that at least one of the living children dies when the mother goes for sterilization. But despite these, women long for sterilization. The reason being simple that modern temporary contraceptive methods, especially condoms and pills, demand correct knowledge and consistent use, failing which unintended pregnancies result. And it is because of these reasons that women find rescue in sterilization and argue that for the better care of children and family they have to undergo sterilization, otherwise who will feed their children. And in these circumstances, God will forgive us!

It means that in popular common sense sterilization is not considered ethical, and both the religious groups have a similar approach. But it is the Muslim reluctance that has been used to highlight and solidify the argument that Muslims do not go for family planning and that they have high fertility. It is here that the popular common sense on Muslim marriage, fertility and family planning needs to be demystified and countered.

CONCLUSION

Discrimination and oppression get accentuated around the carefully crafted popular common sense. The popular common sense provides *a view* of reality but presents it as *the view* or the only reality. *The view* provides the cushion to accept the given version as natural and unchangeable. The discussion on reproductive repertoire helps us locate how the biases, blames and stereotyping across gender, region and religion are rampant and running themes on the issues of reproductive health. Women are made to suffer for early marriage, fertility and son birth. Interestingly, many a times women become the bearers of patriarchy and apparently one woman oppresses the other and vicious circle moves on from one generation to another. This is how hegemony works placing the top dog inside the underdog. This is how patriarchy (the hegemonic theme) legitimizes oppression by using women as an instrument of oppression against women themselves. This needs to be demystified to make *sense* of popular common sense. Similar is trajectory in which the popular common sense puts the rural, poor and illiterate population in dim light and stereotyping further increases when it comes to Muslims. But under the cover of popular common sense, we accept discrimination, marginalization and oppression as natural and unchangeable. The key to counter hegemony lies in questioning the *natural* and organizing the people across the issues of critical consciousness.

REFERENCES

Basu, A.M., 1994, *Culture, the Status of Women and Demographic Behaviour: Illustrated with the Case of India*. Oxford: Clarendon Press.

Basu, A.M., 1997, 'The "Politicization" of Fertility to Achieve Non-Demographic Objectives', *Population Studies*, 51(1): 5–18.

Bose, A., 1988, *From Population to People*, 2 vols. Vol. I. New Delhi: B.R. Publishers Corp.

Bose, A., 1995, 'The Family Welfare Programme in India: Changing Paradigm'. In *The Family Welfare Programmes in India*, edited by Hari Mohan Mathur, New Delhi: Vikas Publication House, pp. 176–97.

Bose, A., 2006, *Beyond Demography: Dialogue with People*. New Delhi: B.R. Publishers Corp.

Bumiller, E., 1991, *May You Be the Mother of a Hundred Sons: A Journey Among the Women of India*. New Delhi: Penguin Books.

Census, 2001, *Census of India 2001*. New Delhi: Registrar General of India, Directorate of Census Operations, Government of India.

Census, 2011, *Census of India 2011*. New Delhi: Registrar General of India, Directorate of Census Operations, Government of India.

Datta, P.K., 1999, *Carving Blocs: Communal Ideology in Early Twentieth-Century Bengal*. New Delhi: Oxford University Press.

Endres, M.E., 1975, *On Defusing the Population Bomb*. Cambridge: Mass Halstead Press.

Enke, S., 1966, 'The Economic Aspects of Solving Population Growth', *Economic Journal*, 76: 44–56.

Forgacs, D., 2000 (1988), *The Gramsci Reader: Selected Writings 1916–1935*. New York: New York University Press.

Gramsci, A., 2010 (1971), *Selections from the Prison Notebooks*, edited and translated by Quintin Hoare and Geoffrey Nowell Smith, New Delhi: Orient Blackswan.

International Institute for Population Sciences and Macro International, 2007, *National Family Health Survey (NFHS-3), 2005–06: India*. Mumbai: IIPS.

Ives, P., 2004, *Language & Hegemony in Gramsci*. London: Pluto Press.

Jeffery, P. and R. Jeffery, 2006, *Confronting Saffron Demography: Religion Fertility and Women's Status in India*. Gurgaon: Three Essays.

Kakar, S., 1990 (1989), *Intimate Relations: Exploring Indian Sexuality*. New Delhi: Penguin Books.

Mandelbaum, D.G., 1974, *Human Fertility in India: Social Components and Policy Perspectives*. Berkeley: University of California.

Obermeyer, C.M., 1994, 'Reproductive Choices in Islam: Gender and State in Iran and Tunisia', *Studies in Family Planning*, 25(1): 41–51.

Patel, T., 2006 (1994), *Fertility Behaviour: Population and Society in a Rajasthan Village*, 2nd ed. New Delhi: Oxford University Press.

Pathak, K.B. and B.S. Singh, 1995, 'Fertility Transition in India'. In *The Family Welfare Programmes in India*, edited by Hari Mohan Mathur, New Delhi: Vikas Publication House, pp. 176–97.

Rao, M., 2004, *From Population Control to Reproductive Health: Malthusian Arithmetic*. New Delhi: Sage Publications.

Sen, A., 2006, *Identity and Violence: The Illusion of Destiny*. London: Allen Lane-Penguin Books.

Shariff, A. and A. Razzack, 2006, 'Communal Relations and Social Integration'. In *Social Development Report*, New Delhi: Council for Social Development & Oxford University Press, pp. 96–110.

Wyron, J.B. and J.E. Gordon, 1971, *The Khanna Study: Population Problems in the Rural Punjab*. Cambridge, MA: Harvard University Press.

CHAPTER 8

Maternal Health Care Utilization among Social Groups in Madhya Pradesh

Anil Hiwale and Ajay Choudhary

INTRODUCTION

Equity in health refers to basic level of health security in the form of well-being and services to all social groups of the society. And to understand health inequality, an individual has to grasp the social network between individual mental health and external social environment or relationship. Various studies that have been conducted in India regarding care utilization through household survey show the role of education, information and economic factors as significant. The outcome of a study regarding the role of education on the utilization rates of parental child delivery and postnatal health care reflected that 10 per cent of the women with primary education use maternal health services compared to illiterate women, and 4 per cent avail the exposure of media such as radio, television or printed media for increasing reproductive health care utilization (Shariff and Singh, 2002: 8).

In the Indian context, caste is the most preferential factor to decide the socio-economic conditions. While analysing the caste–class nexus in the context of poverty, it was found that the people below poverty line are none other than SC, ST and other backward classes, and probably it is expressed that these people are living under adverse conditions and poverty. Thus, the health status and utilization of maternal health care could be an indicator to comprehend relationship between health of lower caste and poverty. The study conducted by National Family Health Survey II (NFHS-II) has highlighted the relationship of health attainment with caste in the context of prevalence of anaemia and diarrhoea in women and children especially where these communities have not availed treatment for prevailing diseases due to problem in accessibility and availability of resources related to treatment (Nayar, 2007: 359–60).

Improving the health of individuals, particularly those belonging to socially and economically disadvantaged groups such as scheduled castes and scheduled tribes, is a key objective of the Indian government. The Indian government has embraced the objective of promoting the health of the poor and the disadvantaged in its policy statements and actions, one being its signing of the Alma Ata Declaration of 1978, emphasizing 'Health for All'. In its National Health Policy Statement of 1983, the government stated that 'the highest priority would require being devoted to efforts at launching special programmes for the improvement of maternal and child health, with a special focus on the less privileged sections of society' (Loksabha Secretariat, 1985).

The National Health Policy (NHP), 2002, has set out the basic objective of achieving good health among all populations of the country. The National Common Minimum Programme of the present government has also emphasized on raising public health investment with a special focus on primary health care and increased investment in programmes to improve the reproductive and child health care. It envisages an increase in spending on public health to 2–3 per cent of gross domestic product (GDP) by increased contributions from the central and state governments, and the government has launched the National Rural Health Mission.

Government-sponsored health care facilities function as a three-tier system—sub-centre, Primary Health Centre (PHC) and Community Health Centre (CHC) and cover almost all rural population. In the urban area, state government or municipalities and private health facilities and non-government organizations (NGOs) provide maternal health care. Despite the government's efforts to reach out to pregnant women in all parts of the country to provide all components of maternal health care either for free or for nominal charges, utilization of maternal health remains low in the country. A large proportion of the population lacks access to life-saving obstetric care and utilization of the same is rather low (Maine and Rosenfield, 2001). The institutional delivery is as low as 34 per cent NFHS-3 (2005–06).

There are approximately 170 million pregnancies every year around the world, and every time a woman is pregnant she suddenly risks her life to unpredictable complications that could result in her death or injury and the death or injury of her infant. At least 40 per cent of all pregnant women experience some type of complication during their pregnancies. For about 15 per cent, the complication will be potentially life-threatening and require prompt obstetric care (Koblinsky et al., 1993). About 500,000 women die due to pregnancy-related causes each year (Hill et al., 2001). Maternal death occurs due to the lack of natal care, postnatal care and assistance. Maternal deaths have both direct and indirect causes. About 80 per cent of the maternal deaths are due to direct cause, which include obstetric complications such as severe bleeding, infection, unsafe abortion, hypertensive disorders (eclampsia) and obstructed labour.

Ninety-nine per cent of pregnancy-related deaths occurred in the developing world. A woman's lifetime risk of dying from pregnancy-related complications or during childbirth is 1 in 48 in developing countries versus 1 child in 1800 in the developed world. From a global perspective, India accounts for 19 per cent of all live births worldwide and 27 per cent of all maternal deaths. Maternal deaths account for a considerable proportion of all deaths among women of reproductive age, especially in rural areas. Regional disparities are wide; maternal mortality is estimated to be almost twice as high in the four northern states of Bihar, Madhya Pradesh, Rajasthan and Uttar Pradesh (823 per 100,000 births) than in rest of India (457 per 100,000 births) (Bhat et al., 1992).

Education of women is the most important factor in determining increase in utilization of maternal health care in rural and, more pronouncedly, in urban areas (Becker et al., 1993; Obermeyer, 1993; Bhatia and Cleand, 1995; Govindasamy and Ramesh, 1997; Sivakami and Kulkarni, 2003). Safe motherhood is a human right and must be underpinned by laws and politics that support effective action to increase women's access to basic education, adequate nutrition, economic resources, as well as appropriate health services. In India, more than 100,000 women die every year from the cause related to pregnancy and childbirth. The infant mortality rate in Madhya Pradesh is the third highest among the states of India. The infant mortality in NFHS-3 is estimated to be 70 deaths before the age of one year per 1,000 live births.

Poverty has been observed as the strong linkage with ill health due to limited access to quality of health care and relationship between the status and social relation. The health relations to low social status are potentially harmful to health (Tonovan et al., 2011: 35). It means that socio-economic deprivation and ill health cause serious adverse effects on health. The social and welfare measure in other words is an essential criterion of contribution to comprehend ill health and poverty. Thus, poverty leads to vicious circle, which explains the health inequalities in Indian society. To wipe out this circle, the health care services should be distributed according to health needs of individuals as per socio-economic characteristic. Illiteracy, coupled with poverty and severe deprivation among the people of this group, has given rise to all kinds of health problems. A solution to these problems in general lies in improving the general socio-economic conditions of these underprivileged groups. Government has to stress more on strategy to increase their capabilities and empowerment by facilitating their education and health care. Health facilities do exist, but utilization is not there perhaps because of the lack of awareness and indifference among the people about government health facilities (Ram et al., 1997).

ASPECT OF THE STUDY

From an ethical and human rights perspective, narrowing avoidable disparities in health is imperative. Inequalities in health are pervasive within state and among social groups. Even in states where aggregate health indicators are improving, some health gaps between population groups are widening or remaining stagnant. The size and dynamics of these gaps vary considerably among social groups.

Caste and religion are intertwined with every aspect of life in India. Hinduism is the largest religion that has been further divided into different caste groups broadly termed as scheduled castes (SCs), scheduled tribes (STs), other backward classes (OBCs) and others. According to 2001 Census, the SCs constitute 15.17 per cent, the SCs account for 20.27 per cent and others constitute 64.56 per cent in Madhya Pradesh. According to the NFHS-III, 18 per cent of household head belong to SCs, 21 per cent belong to STs, 40 per cent belong to OBCs and 21 per cent belong to other castes in Madhya Pradesh. The Constitution of India guarantees social, economic and political provisions for protection and promotion of interest of SCs, STs, OBCs and minorities. In order to bring them at par with the rest of the society by adopting the approach of social justice to ensure equal rights, access to public services and resources to enable them to develop their potential and capacities as agents of social change, through the process of planned development. In view of the above discussion, this paper is undertaken to study the maternal health utilization by residence, educational level and wealth index among social groups in Madhya Pradesh.

METHODOLOGY AND DATA INTERPRETATION

It has been analysed from NFHS conducted in 2005–06 (NFHS-3). In Madhya Pradesh, NFHS-3 collected information from a representative sample of 5,488 households for urban and rural areas. NFHS-3 interviewed 6,427 women of age 15–49 years from all the selected households and 2,725 men of age 15–54 years from a sub-sample of household to obtain information on population, health and nutrition in the state. In this paper, bivariate analysis has been used to study the utilization of maternal health care among social groups. The full antenatal care (ANC) refers to three or more antenatal check-ups, at least two TT injections and taken at least 90 iron and folic acid tablets/syrup.

SOCIAL BACKGROUND OF THE WOMEN AMONG SOCIAL GROUPS IN MADHYA PRADESH

The per cent distribution of women among social groups in Madhya Pradesh by background characteristics is presented in Table 8.1.

Out of 6,427 women, majority of the women belong to rural areas among all the social groups. The highest 95 per cent of the women among STs followed by 77 per cent among OBCs, 71 per cent among SCs and lowest, 58 per cent, among other category lives in rural areas. The percentage of women living in urban areas is highest, 42 per cent, among other category and lowest, 5 per cent, among the ST category. The percentage of non-educated women is highest, 79 per cent, among the ST category; whereas the percentage of primary educated is highest, 22 per cent, among women of the OBC category. The 45 per cent and 11 per cent of the women among other castes are secondary and higher secondary educated, respectively. The highest 94 per cent of women among STs and lowest 32 per cent among other castes belongs to poor wealth index category. The highest 18 per cent of women among the OBC category and lowest 4 per cent among the

Table 8.1 Percent Distribution of Social Groups by Background Characteristics in Madhya Pradesh, 2005–06

	Types of Social Groups			
Background Characteristics	*SC*	*ST*	*OBC*	*Others*
Place of Residence				
Rural	70.6	94.6	77.3	57.7
Urban	29.4	5.4	22.7	42.3
Educational Level				
No education	58.7	78.9	53.0	31.8
Primary	19.4	12.8	21.7	12.5
Secondary	19.2	8.3	22.8	44.9
Higher	2.7	*	2.5	10.8
Wealth Index				
Poor	68.3	93.8	62.9	32.4
Middle	13.2	4.4	17.8	16.7
Rich	18.4	1.8	19.4	50.9
Exposure to Mass Media				
No exposure	61.3	70.2	57.3	49.6
Exposure	38.7	29.8	42.7	50.4
Occupation of Husband				
Services	12.9	3.4	16.1	37.3
Agricultural employee	34.1	51.9	44.0	32.4
Un-skilled, skilled manual	53.0	44.7	39.9	30.3

Note: * Less frequency.

ST category belongs to middle wealth index category, whereas the highest 51 per cent women among other castes and lowest 2 per cent women among STs belong to the rich category. The highest 50 per cent of the women among other castes followed by 43 per cent women among OBCs, 39 per cent women among SCs and lowest 30 per cent women among STs are exposed to mass media. The highest 37 per cent are working in service sector in case of the husbands of other caste women, 44 per cent are working in agriculture in case of the husbands of OBC women and 53 per cent are working as unskilled/skilled manual labour in case of the husbands of SC women.

ANTENATAL CARE UTILIZATION AMONG SOCIAL GROUPS IN MADHYA PRADESH

All women need additional care during pregnancy. They need to eat and rest more when they are pregnant. All women must be given TT injection and the full course of iron folic acid tablets. All women need to be oriented properly and prepare them for delivery process. The percentage of ANC utilization among social groups in Madhya Pradesh is presented in Table 8.2.

Table 8.2 Maternal Health Care Utilization among Social Groups in Madhya Pradesh, 2005–06

	Types of Social Groups				
Maternal Utilization	*SC*	*ST*	*OBC*	*Others*	*Total*
TT Injection					
Never	16.0	37.5	12.0	7.7	18.2
Partial (<2)	13.1	10.7	12.0	8.0	11.2
Full (<2)	70.9	51.7	76.1	84.3	70.6
Iron Tablets Taken					
Never	6.9	5.2	8.3	7.3	7.19
Partial (<89)	74.5	80.4	74.4	61.5	73.15
Full (<90)	18.6	14.4	17.3	31.3	19.66
ANC Visits					
Never	17.5	36.5	16.7	10.0	20.5
Partial (<3)	44.4	37.6	39.6	32.6	38.8
Full (<3)	38.1	25.9	43.8	57.3	40.7
Levels of full ANC use					
Never	0.0	0.6	0.0	0.0	0.6
Partial	89.2	93.8	89.3	75.9	87.8
Full	10.8	5.6	10.7	24.1	12.0
Place of Delivery					
Home	74.4	91.6	72.3	47.1	73.5
Institution	25.3	8.1	27.5	52.5	26.2
Others (NGO, etc.)	0.3	0.4	0.2	0.4	0.3

The percentage of women given TT injection is 71 per cent in Madhya Pradesh, and it varies from highest 84 per cent among women of other castes to lowest 52 per cent among women of STs.

The percentage of women given partial TT injection is highest 13 per cent among women of SCs and lowest 8 per cent among women of other castes. The percentage of women who had never taken TT injection is 18 per cent in Madhya Pradesh, and it varies from highest 38 per cent among women of STs to lowest 8 per cent among women of other castes. The percentage of women who had taken 90 or more than 90 tablets is 20 per cent in Madhya Pradesh, and it varies from highest 31 per cent among women of other castes to lowest 14 per cent among women of STs. The percentage of women who had taken partial iron folic acid tablets is 74 per cent in Madhya Pradesh, and it is highest 80 per cent among women of STs and lowest 62 per cent among women of other castes. The percentage of women who had never taken iron folic acid tablets is 21 per cent in Madhya Pradesh, and it varies from highest 37 per cent among women of STs to lowest 10 per cent among women of other castes. The 41 per cent of women had full antenatal visits during pregnancy, and it varies from highest 57 per cent among women of other castes to lowest 26 per cent of women among the ST category. The 39 per cent of women in Madhya Pradesh had partial ANC visits during pregnancy, and it varies from highest 44 per cent of women among STs to 33 per cent of women among other castes. The 21 per cent of women never gone for ANC visit during pregnancy, and it is highest 37 per cent of women among STs and lowest 10 per cent of women among other castes. The percentage of women who had availed full ANC is 12 per cent in Madhya Pradesh, and it varies from highest 24 per cent of women among other castes and lowest 6 per cent of women among STs. The percentage of women who had partially availed ANC is 88 per cent in Madhya Pradesh, and it varies from highest 94 per cent of women among STs and lowest 76 per cent of women among other castes. Nearly, three-fourth of women delivered at homes and one-fourth delivered in institutions. The percentage of home delivery varies from highest 92 per cent of women among STs to lowest 47 per cent of women among other castes. The percentage of women who had institutional delivery is highest 53 per cent of women among other castes and lowest 8 per cent of women among STs. The percentage of women who had delivered at other places is < 1 per cent among all the social groups. The postnatal check-ups performed by doctors is 13 per cent, by ANMs is 63 per cent, by other health personnels is 4 per cent and by *Dai*/trained birth attendants is 20 per cent.

MATERNAL HEALTH CARE UTILIZATION AMONG SOCIAL GROUPS BY RESIDENCE

The maternal health care utilization among social groups by place of residence is shown in Table 8.3.

Table 8.3 Maternal Health Care Utilization among Social Groups by Place of Residence in Madhya Pradesh, 2005–06

			Place of Delivery		
Place of Residence	*Types of Social Groups*	*Full ANC Use*	*Home Delivery*	*Institution*	*Others*
Rural	SC	6.7	85.9	14.1	0.0
	ST	5.0	92.8	6.8	0.4
	OBC	8.9	79.5	20.3	0.3
	Others	16.8	62.1	37.9	0.0
Urban	SC	19.8	46.8	52.1	1.1
	ST	17.6	68.9	31.1	0.0
	OBC	15.9	47.6	52.4	0.0
	Others	32.0	26.5	72.6	0.9

It can be seen from table that the utilization of full ANC is higher in urban areas as compared to rural areas among all the social groups. In rural area, the use of full ANC varies from highest 17 per cent among women of other castes to lowest 5 per cent of women among women of STs. The use of full ANC varies from highest 32 per cent of women among other castes to lowest 16 per cent of women among OBCs. The percentage of home delivery is higher in rural areas and lower in urban areas among social groups. The percentage of home delivery is higher among SC and ST women than OBC and other caste women in rural areas, whereas the percentage of home delivery is higher among ST women than OBC, SC and other caste women in urban areas. This shows that there is a gap between utilization of maternal health care in rural and urban areas and rural areas lagging behind urban areas. In case of social groups, ST and SC are lagging behind OBC and other castes in utilization of maternal health care services.

MATERNAL HEALTH CARE UTILIZATION AMONG SOCIAL GROUPS BY EDUCATION

All pregnant women need periodic health check-ups so that maternal complications or risk factors are identified in time, treatment is started early and the women are motivated to have safe delivery by the trained staffs or to deliver at the sub-centre or PHC. They are expected to visit health facilities to have at least three antenatal check-ups for blood, blood pressure and urine check-up and other procedures to detect pregnancy-related complications to avoid the maternal death and infant death during delivery. The maternal health care utilization among social groups in Madhya Pradesh is summarized in Table 8.4.

Table 8.4 Percentage of Maternal Health Care Utilization among Social Groups by Education in Madhya Pradesh, 2005–06

Education Level	*Types of Social Groups*	*Full ANC*	*Place of Delivery*		
			Home Delivery	*Institutional*	*Others*
No Education	SC	5.9	82.3	17.7	0.0
	ST	5.8	93.3	6.2	0.4
	OBC	5.7	83.2	16.5	0.3
	Others	8.8	69.8	30.2	0.0
Primary	SC	8.8	78.0	22.0	0.0
	ST	3.6	84.5	15.5	0.0
	OBC	11.0	66.4	32.9	0.7
	Others	18.4	65.7	34.3	0.0
Secondary	SC	18.8	54.5	43.9	1.6
	ST	6.8	84.5	15.5	0.0
	OBC	15.5	58.0	42.0	0.0
	Others	23.8	37.1	62.0	0.8
Higher	SC	53.8	17.6	82.4	0.0
	ST	*	*	*	*
	OBC	52.9	17.6	82.4	0.0
	Others	57.4	0.0	100.0	0.0

Note: * Less frequency.

The full ANC by education varies among social groups. The full ANC is lowest among non-educated and primary educated women as compared to secondary and higher secondary educated women among all social groups. The full ANC is lower among women of SCs and STs as compared to women of OBCs and other castes. According to the education level, the full ANC utilization is lowest among women of OBC as compare to SC, ST and other castes in case of non-educated women. In case of primary educated women, the OBC and other caste women had availed higher full ANC as compared to SC and ST women. The per cent of full ANC by secondary education is higher among women of other castes and SC as compared to OBC and ST and the per cent of full ANC by higher secondary education is higher among women of other castes and SC as compared to OBC. The per cent of full ANC by primary education varies from only 3.6 per cent of women among ST to 8.8 per cent of women among SC, 11 per cent of women among OBC and 18.4 per cent of the women in other category. In case of women with secondary education again ST is in worst condition. Only 6.8 per cent of women among ST received full ANC, and this percentage is 18.4 per cent of women among SC, 15.5 per cent of women among OBC and 23.8 per cent of women among other castes. The percentage of full ANC by higher education of women is 53.8 per cent among SC, 52.9 per cent among OBC and 57.4 per cent among other castes. This indicates that there are variations in utilization of full ANC by education among social groups.

The percentage of women who had home delivery is highest among non-educated, whereas the percentage of institutional delivery is highest among educated women. In case of non-educated groups, the ST women had highest 93 per cent of home delivery and it is 82 per cent for SC, 83 per cent for OBC and 70 per cent for other castes. In case of women with primary education, again ST is having highest 84.5 per cent of home delivery followed by 78 per cent of women among SC, 66 per cent of women among OBC and lowest 66 per cent of women among other castes. In case of highly educated women, the percentage of institutional deliveries are higher and home deliveries are lower than the primary and non-educated women.

MATERNAL HEALTH CARE UTILIZATION AMONG SOCIAL GROUPS BY WEALTH INDEX

The percentage of maternal health care utilization by wealth index is presented in Table 8.5. Full ANC by wealth index of the household of the women is found to be highest in case of rich wealth index followed by medium wealth index and lowest among poor wealth index. The use of full ANC is found to be higher among other castes and OBC than SC and ST. The home delivery is found to be higher among the women of poor health index, whereas institutional delivery is higher in case of rich health index. In case of social groups, the percentage of home

Table 8.5 Percentage of Maternal Health Care Utilization among Social Groups by Wealth Index in Madhya Pradesh, 2005–06

Wealth Index	*Types of Social Groups*	*Full ANC Use*	*Place of Delivery*		
			Home	*Institutional*	*Others*
Poor					
	SC	6.3	87.1	12.9	0.0
	ST	5.5	92.5	7.1	0.4
	OBC	5.6	83.2	16.4	0.3
	Others	10.8	77.4	22.6	0.0
Middle					
	SC	20.0	64.3	35.7	*
	ST	0.0	78.9	21.1	*
	OBC	15.3	66.7	33.3	*
	Others	11.4	49.5	50.5	*
Rich					
	SC	21.5	34.2	64.1	1.7
	ST	16.7	73.3	26.7	0.0
	OBC	20.4	41.8	58.2	0.0
	Others	33.3	26.7	72.6	0.7

Note: * Less frequency.

delivery is higher among SC and ST than OBC and other castes among the women of poor wealth index. In case of medium and rich wealth index, the percentage of home delivery is higher among ST and OBC than SC and other castes, whereas the percentage of institutional delivery is higher among SC and other castes than ST and OBC. This indicates that there are differentials in the utilization of maternal health care among social and economic groups.

SUMMARY AND CONCLUSIONS

The analysis revealed that the utilization of full ANC is very low as compared to use of partial ANC in Madhya Pradesh and it varies among social groups. The utilization of maternal health care is lower in rural areas than urban areas and SC, ST and OBC women are lagging behind the other caste women in utilization of health services. The full ANC by education varies among social groups. The full ANC is lowest among non-educated and primary educated women as compared to secondary and higher secondary educated women among all social groups. The full ANC is lower among women of SCs and STs as compared to women of OBCs and other castes. Full ANC by wealth index of the household of the women is found to be highest in case of rich wealth index followed by medium wealth index and lowest among poor wealth index. The use of full ANC is found to be higher among other castes and OBC than SC and ST. Illiteracy coupled with poverty among the SC, ST and OBC groups resulted in lower utilization of maternal health care in Madhya Pradesh. A solution to the problems in general lies in improving the general socio-economic conditions of these underprivileged groups. Government has to stress more on strategy to increase their capabilities and empowerment by facilitating their education and health care.

REFERENCES

Becker, S., H.P. David, H.G. Ronald, G. Connie and E.B. Robert, 1993, 'The Determinants of Use of Maternal and Child Health Services in Metro Cebu, the Philippines', *Health Transition Review*, 3(1): 77–89.

Bhatia, J.C. and J. Cleland, 1995, 'Determinants of Maternal Care in a Region of South India', *Health Transition Review*, 5(2): 127–42.

Govindasamy, P. and B.M. Ramesh, 1997, 'Maternal Education and Utilization of Maternal and Child Health Services in India', *NFHS Survey Subject Reports No.5*. Mumbai: International Institute for Population Sciences.

Hill, K., C. AbouZahr and T. Wardlaw, 2001, 'Estimates of Maternal Mortality for 1995', *Bulletin of the World Health Organization*, 79(3): 182–93.

Koblinsky, M.A., O.M.R. Campbell and D. Harlow, 1993, 'Mother and More: A Broader Perspective on Women's Health'. In *The Health of Women: A Global Perspective*, edited by M. Koblinsky, J. Timyan and J. Gay, Oxford: Westview Press.

Loksabha Secretariat, 1985, *National Health Policy*. New Delhi: Loksabha Secretariat.

Maine, D. and A. Rosenfield, 2001, 'The AMDD Program: History, Focus and Structure', *International Journal of Gynecology & Obstetrics*, 74(2): 99–103.

Mari Bhat, P.N., K. Navaneetham and S. Irudaya Rajan, 1992, *Maternal Mortality in India: Eestimates from an Econometric Model*, Population Research Centre, Dharwad: Working Paper 24 (January).

National Health Policy (NHP), 2002, 'Ministry of Health and Family Welfare', Department of Health and Family Welfare, Government of India, [online] available at http://mohfw.nic.in/

Nayar, K.R., 2007, 'Social Exclusion, Caste and Health: A Review Based on the Social Determinants Framework', *Indian Journal of Medical Research*, 126: 355–63.

Obermeyer, C.M., 1993, 'Maternal Health Care and Women's Status: A Comparison of Morocco and Tunisia', *Studies in Family Planning*, 24(6): 354–65.

Ram, F., K.B. Pathak and K.I. Annamma, 1997, 'Utilization of Health Care Services by the Under Privileged Section of Population in India', *IASSI Quarterly*, 16(3–4).

Shariff, Abusaleh and Geeta Singh, 2002, 'Determinants of Maternal Health Care Utilization in India: Evidences from a Recent Household Survey', *National Council of Applied Economic Research*, February.

Sivakami, M. and P.M. Kulkarni, 2003, 'Are Socially and Economically Weaker Sections Deprived of Maternal Health Care in Tamil Nadu?' *Journal of Health and Population in Developing Countries*, [online] available at http://www.jhpdc.unc.edu.

Tonovan, Tamara, Michael Sauer and Frank Schulz-Nieswandt, 2011, *Growth, Inequality, Poverty and Pro-Poor Health Policy* (*Gesundheitsokonomie: Politik und Management*), vol. 7. London: LIT Verlag Munster Publication.

WHO, 2004, *Maternal Mortality in 1996*. Geneva: WHO.

WHO, UNICEF and UNFP, 2000, *Maternal Mortality Report in 2000*. Geneva: WHO.

Part III

Diversities and Deprivations: Maternal Health Contextualized

CHAPTER 9

Reproductive Health and Developmental Needs of Adolescent Girls in Manipur

Thounaojam Sunitibala Devi

INTRODUCTION

Adolescence is a modern cultural and social phenomenon, and therefore the ages of adolescents vary by culture. There is still a debate going on the age of adolescence that is what age adolescence begins and when it emerges into adulthood as the time span is not the same for every person. The World Health Organization (WHO) defines adolescence in terms of both age between 10 and 19 years and a phase of life marked by special developmental attributes such as rapid physical growth and development, physical, social and psychological maturity, but not all at same time, sexual maturity and the onset of sexual activity, experimentation, development of adult identity, transition from total socio-independence (WHO, 2005). The United Nations Population Fund (UNFPA) has also given the age of adolescents as 10–19 years. In contrast, in the United States, adolescence is generally considered to begin between the ages of 12 and 14 years, and to end at the ages of 19 or 20 years. As distinct from adolescence, the word 'teenager' is more easily defined as a person who is 13–19 years of age. In the Report of the Working Group, the Government of India, Planning Commission, June 2001, the working group for the Tenth Five-Year Plan has accepted age of adolescents from 10–19 years. Again, the Government of India in its document on Youth Policy (2003) defines adolescence as 13–19 years age group. Thus, the only universal definition of adolescence is to mark it as a period in which a person is no longer a child and not yet an adult.

Adolescence is a period of rapid growth, development and change. Numerous changes take place, which are of vital importance in conditioning the behaviour and thinking of adolescents. This period of transition is characterized by a combination of physical, psychological and social changes. Generally, adolescence is a period of transition from puberty to adulthood. Puberty refers to the period of physical growth and the development of secondary sexual characteristics.

It is a known fact that girls begin their pubertal development and attain full growth at an earlier age than boys. Girls grow faster in height and weight at approximately 12 years of age; whereas in the case of boys, it is approximately at 14 years of age (Tanner, 1972). Young girls become aware of the physical changes taking place, and this deeply affects their thinking. Most of them develop some new feelings, which are very hard for them to understand. Menstruation may be a very upsetting event for some girls who are not prepared for it. Young girls become self-conscious about their development if they believe their growth is not normal. This happens with those girls who mature late and when they are not growing as their friends. This is also true of those girls who mature early. They are taller and more developed sexually. This makes them feel awkward and self-conscious about their appearance because the girls are different from their pubertal friends (Rice, 1990).

Most researchers have pointed out that girls are more concerned than boys about their physical appearance. They are concerned about the size and shape of their breast, the dress they wear and other accessories. Tallness, pressure to remain thin, menstruation, underweight, defective teeth, defective speech and shortness are some of the major problems of concern for adolescent girls (Cole, 1962). Because of this, early maturing girls are known to have more problems that are emotional, a lower self-image and higher rates of depression, anxiety and disordered eating (Ge et al., 1996). This deeply affected their interests, their social behaviour and the quality of their affective life (Blos, 1962). The evidence suggests that bodily changes play an important role in the overall development of adolescents.

This period of transition is also regarded as very crucial. Some young girls are unaware about menstruation and the physical changes that have taken place. They are not informed about it, thus they lack knowledge on the biological processes of maturation and normal physiology. As discussion on sexuality is absent in the Indian society, young girls are not prepared mentally for the changes. Thus, they have psychological problems, which may deteriorate their health condition. This is true more in case of young girls in a socially and economically backward family where discrimination is high. They are deprived of the attention and care that they needed most, therefore they are a burden to their families and have poor self-image as compared to their brothers.

Another important factor for psychological stress among adolescent girls is the onset of menstruation. Those young girls, who are not given information about menstruation prior to its onset, were frightened at the sight of blood for the first time. They are also vulnerable to infections if prior information about hygienic practices regarding menstruation is not given. In Western societies, 'it is argued that menarche conveys conflicting societal messages, it represents the beginning of womanhood and sexuality, but girls of this age are seen as too young to be sexually active' (Wichstrom, 1999). In the Indian society, menstruation is considered a polluting factor among Hindus. There are certain myths and taboos associated with menstruation. A menstruating girl/woman is restricted from cooking food, from touching anything in the kitchen or visit temple. While the girls/women are very knowledgeable about the myths and taboos, they have little knowledge about the biological processes of maturation and normal physiology (Shukla, 2005).

Thus, young girls lack information on hygienic practice during menstruation, which consequently may increase susceptibility to various infections. In a study of ICMR, it was found that knowledge and awareness about puberty, menstruation, physical changes, reproduction, contraception, pregnancy, childbearing, reproductive tract infections (RTIs), sexually transmitted infections (STIs) and HIV was low among young adolescents in the 10–14 year age group (ICMR, 1992). Young girls in this age group are unaware and are not informed about menstruation prior to its onset. However, the study showed that the older age group (15–19 years) had better knowledge.

In a poor socially disadvantaged family, the period of adolescence for a young girl is for a limited period. This is because of the prevalence of gender discrimination and low socio-economic status where the preference for son is high. Discrimination starts right from the birth of a female child. From lineage to religion and from appropriating a hefty dowry to earning for the family, everything points towards begetting a son, which leads to the practice of female foeticide.

Thus, the health and well-being of adolescents—the future parents are very important. However, the importance of adolescents' health and of nutrition is recognized recently. Adolescents make roughly 20 per cent of the total world population, of whom 85 per cent live in developing countries (WHO, UNFPA, UNICEF, 1995). India has an estimated 200 million adolescents' population (CEDPA, 2001). About one-fifth of India's population is in the adolescent age group of 10–19 years (Census of India, 2001). Adolescents constitute a sizeable proportion of the Indian mothers. Despite the huge growing adolescents' population, the health needs of adolescents have neither been researched nor addressed adequately; particularly, their reproductive health needs are often misunderstood, unrecognized or underestimated. Policies and programmes in India focused little on the health of adolescents as they are basically considered a healthy group having the lowest mortality and morbidity compared with other age groups.

Keeping all these aspects in mind, in this paper, an attempt has been made to examine adolescent girls' level of awareness, the problems and reactions regarding menstruation and physical changes that have taken place due to the onset of puberty.

METHODOLOGY

This study is exploratory cum diagnostic in nature. The study is based on both primary and secondary sources of data. Selection of universe in terms of area and in terms of the respondents has been done by adopting multi-stage random sampling. In terms of area, Imphal East and Imphal West districts of Manipur state have been selected for the purpose of study. A semi-structured interview schedule is used to collect data from unmarried adolescent girls. The total sample size consists of 300 respondents.

The semi-structured interview schedule consisted of independent and dependent variables such as age, religion, educational background, awareness regarding physical changes occurred in their bodies, etc.

RESULTS AND DISCUSSION

Profile of Respondents

The average age of respondents is 15 years, majority are Hindus and all of them are educated (Table 9.1). About 40 per cent respondents

Table 9.1 Distribution of Respondents by Selected Background Characteristics

Total Respondents = 300

Characteristics	*Number (%)*
Age	
11–13	66 (22)
14–16	138 (46)
17–19	96 (32)
Religion	
Hinduism	174 (23)
Meiteism	69 (58)
Christianity	27 (9)
Islam	30 (10)
Levels of education	
Primary	0 (0)
High school	153 (51)
Secondary	93 (31)
Under graduates	54 (18)
Parent's treatment towards their children	
Received differential treatment	120 (40)
Received equal treatment	180 (60)

Note: Figures in parenthesis are in per cent. The same will be applicable to all the tables presented in the study.

revealed having received differential treatment from their parents. What is revealed and interesting to know is that all the respondents 100 per cent helped their parents in the household responsibilities while not all the respondents' brother do so (Table 9.1). However, more than half of the brothers of the respondents helped their parents in the household responsibilities. Girls' work responsibilities at home often increase as they get older. One important finding is that no discrimination in terms of education, food, etc. can be seen. Although young girls are not always deprived of the attention and care they needed most, they are often found to be regarded a burden on their families and have poor self-image as compared to their brothers. Adolescent girls have been mainly socialized to care for others rather than themselves. They feel that whatever is happening is natural and so as always expected, they help their parents in the household chores while it is not always so in case of their brothers.

Menstruation: Awareness and Reaction of Respondents towards Menstruation

With the lack of information, the first menstrual flow can be terrifying to a young girl. In most parts of India, the first menstrual experience is often a traumatic and very negative experience for young girls (George, 1994). Negative responses such as shame, fear, anxiety and depression are most common. It has been found that menarche emerged as the strongest predictor of depression and anxiety among adolescent girls (Patton et al., 1996). Most young girls suffered from physical discomforts, increased emotions and mood changes and disruption of activities and social life. Some accepted menstruation in a natural way because they have been taught about it. Thus, the reaction to menstruation depends on awareness and knowledge about it.

As shown in Table 9.2, it is found that the age of first menstruation ranges from 10–14 years with maximum number of respondents at 13 years of age. It clearly shows that awareness about menstruation prior to its onset is high. Maximum 78 per cent of the respondents have knowledge about menstruation, whereas the rest 22 per cent respondents have no prior knowledge and their problems need to be seriously addressed. The data show that respondents are having the required information, which is very important, as adolescence is a period of change, namely physical, mental, etc. Here, mothers play the most important role in giving knowledge regarding menstruation to the young girls.

Menstruation is regarded as an important factor for psychological stress among adolescent girls because it may be very upsetting event for some girls who are not prepared for it. The result shows this fact also, those girls who are not given prior information before its onset do suffer from psychological stress, for example, they complained to suffer from discomfort, disgust and are even scared to see blood flow for the first time. This problem if not looked into in time may create further health problems to the young girls. It is therefore,

Table 9.2 Distribution of Respondents by Awareness and Reaction towards Menstruation

Total Respondents = 300

Responses	*Number (%)*
Age at menarche	
10	6 (2)
11	45 (15)
12	96 (32)
13	144 (48)
14	9 (3)
Reaction to first menstruation	
Suffer from mental stress	165 (55)
Face no problem	135 (45)
Awareness on menstruation	
Aware	234 (78)
Unaware	66 (22)
Source of information on menstruation	
Mother	153 (51)
Sister	42 (14)
Friends	27 (9)
Books	12 (4)
Unaware	66 (22)

necessary to give young girls the knowledge and information about menstruation prior to menarche.

Menstrual Practices and Restrictions Faced by Respondents during Menstruation

Adolescent girls are vulnerable to infections if prior information about hygienic practices regarding menstruation is not given. There are certain myths and taboos associated with menstruation. While the girls are very knowledgeable about the myths and taboos, they have little knowledge about the biological processes of maturation and normal physiology. However, good number of them are found following certain myths that forbid them from taking nutritional food they need to take during menstruation.

Table 9.3 Distribution of Respondents by Menstrual Practices and Restrictions Faced during Menstruation

Total Respondents = 300

Responses	*Number (%)*
Material used during menstruation	
Sanitary pads/napkins	171 (57)
Cloth	129 (43)
Restricted from performing religious rituals	
Yes	207 (69)
No	93 (31)
Restricted from touching religious items, kitchen ware, cooking, etc.	
Yes	216 (72)
No	84 (28)
Reactions of respondents towards restrictions	
Suffer from mental stress	93 (31)
No problem	207 (69)

To add to this, young girls also lack information on hygienic practice during menstruation, which consequently may increase susceptibility to various infections. It is clear from the Table 9.3 that maximum number of young girls (57 per cent) used readymade sanitary napkins/pads during menstruation and 43 per cent respondents used cloth, the traditional way. One reason is that most of the respondents are still unaware of the consequences of using unhygienic cloth during menstruation. This problem needs to be seriously dealt with. Another reason is the high cost of sanitary pads that some of the girls cannot afford to buy one. Very unhygienic practice that can be seen is that some of the respondents reused the old cloth. The practice is to wash the used cloth with detergent and keep it in a secret place for next menstruation. Sometimes to avoid from the sight of male members in the family, they kept it in a very unhygienic place, which may eventually create gynaecological problems such as urinary tract infections to the young girls.

Table 9.4 Distribution of Respondents by Awareness and Reaction towards Physical Change

Total Respondents = 300

Responses	*Number (%)*
Awareness on physical changes	
Aware	135 (45)
Unaware	165 (55)
Source of information	
Mother	63 (21)
Friends	24 (8)
Sisters	42 (14)
Books	6 (2)
Unaware of change	165 (55)

The young girls have several restrictions to be followed during menstruation. They are not allowed to perform religious rituals, not allowed to touch religious items and are also restricted from cooking for the family. Some are even restricted from washing hair, taking a bath, etc. Such restrictions make the condition of the young girls worse because they have to suffer from embarrassment when all the family members including male members come to know about their situation. The table indicates that 69 per cent of the respondents are restricted from performing any religious rituals while 31 per cent of respondents do not have any such problems. About 72 per cent respondents are also restricted from touching religious items, kitchenware, cooking, etc., whereas about 28 per cent of the respondents do not face such kind of restrictions.

Awareness and Reaction of Respondents towards Physical Change

Another important factor for psychological stress among adolescent girls is the lack of knowledge on physical change that has taken place due to the onset of puberty. Adolescence is a time of rapid physical development and deep emotional changes. Most young girls often lack knowledge on the various changes that have taken place in them, hence they face overwhelming problems. The changes can be more worrying to some girls, especially to those who are shy and who do not like to ask questions. Young people of this age begin to think and feel differently. Relationship with friends starts to be much closer, whereas relationships within the family change. They become very emotional and conscious about their appearance. Researchers in their studies have observed that adolescent girls experienced greater stress and are twice as likely to be depressed, attempt suicide four or five times as often, as compared to boys (Debold, 1995). The reason for girl's depression has been found to be linked to negative feelings about their bodies and appearances.

The respondents' level of awareness regarding the physiological changes is found to be not that high (45 per cent), shown in Table 9.4. More than half of the girls (55 per cent) are unaware and uninformed about the physical changes. Bodily changes play an important role in the overall development of adolescents. But, parents (mothers only 21 per cent) who are regarded as the most important source of information for their children fail to prove. Here, we can see clearly the communication gap between the parents and their children. As discussion on sexuality is absent in Manipuri society, young girls are not prepared mentally for the physical changes. Thus, they (59 per cent) began to have psychological problems, such as, they were emotional, had a lower self-image and suffered from depression, anxiety and disordered eating, etc. This deeply affected their interests, their social behaviour and the quality of their affective life, which may deteriorate their health condition and may have long-lasting effect.

Awareness of Respondents Regarding Contraception, Pregnancy and Childbirth, STDs, RTIs and HIV/AIDS

AIDS prevention may largely depend on health education and behavioural changes based on their awareness on contraception, pregnancy, childbirth, RTIs, STIs, HIV/AIDS, etc., particularly among the young girls who are more prone to risky behaviour. Lack of access to correct information, tendency to experiment and an environment that makes discussing issues around sexuality a taboo add to their vulnerability to the devastating AIDS epidemic (Timothy and Rajan, 2004). Young women are said to be biologically more vulnerable to HIV infection than young men—a situation aggravated by their lack of access to information on HIV and even lesser power to exercise control over their sexual lives. Early marriage also poses special risks to young people, particularly women. This is especially relevant for India, where a majority of the girls are married off by the time they are 18 years of age.

Table 9.5 Distribution of Respondents by Awareness Regarding Contraception, Pregnancy Childbirth, STDs, RTIs, and HIV/AIDS

Total Respondents = 300

Responses	*Number (%)*
Awareness regarding contraception, pregnancy and childbirth	
Aware	204 (68)
Unaware	96 (32)
Awareness regarding STDs, RTIs and HIV/AIDS	
Aware	204 (68)
Unaware	96 (32)

Table 9.5 shows that a majority (68 per cent) of the respondents are aware about the various available contraception, pregnancy and childbearing. However, though majority of the respondents are having awareness, 32 per cent are not aware at all, and this is a matter of great concern. This reveals that a good number of adolescent girls in Manipur are still ignorant of the information that are regarded important or a must before they move into a stage of life, that is, reproduction so as to protect themselves from various risk-taking behaviours and reproductive health problems which if not dealt with in time may last a lifetime. Risk-taking behaviour is considered by some to be a normal part of adolescent development. During adolescence, young people experience great and rapid changes—in their bodies, concerns, relationships and roles in society. Adolescents are also said to gain more independence and begin to experiment with new behaviours; some of which placed them at risk for potentially negative health consequences.

A perusal of Table 9.5 shows that 64 per cent respondents have knowledge regarding RTIs, STIs and HIV/AIDS while 36 per cent are unaware of it. Although the awareness level is high, the remaining group who do not have idea on the said terms may prove to be a growing threat for the spread of STDs, RTIs and HIV/AIDS.

CONCLUSION

Adolescent girls constitute the most important stage in a woman's life, and they form the initial reproductive age group. As preference for a male child is prevalent in Manipuri society, discrimination against girls can be seen in some form or the other. Young girls reveal getting differential treatment from their parents as compared with their brothers. It is also interesting to know that majority of girls are aware of the onset of menstruation, and mothers play an important role in giving the said information. But there are also girls who lack knowledge on the said thing, who were frightened at the sight of blood for the first time and who do suffer from stress. Further, it is shocking to know that some girls are found following unhygienic practices and certain myths during menstruation, which consequently may increase susceptibility to various infections. Another shocking revelation is that more than half of the girls are unaware and uninformed about the physical changes. As discussion on sexuality is absent in Manipuri society, we can clearly see the communication gap between the parents and their children. Therefore, young girls are not prepared mentally for the physical changes and thus suffer from stress. This deeply affected their interests, their social behaviour and the quality of their affective life, which may deteriorate their health condition and may a have long-lasting effect. It also comes to light that girls have knowledge on contraception, pregnancy, childbirth, RTIs, STIs, HIV/AIDS, etc., but still a good number of them are ignorant that may prove to be risky for their future health, if their needs are not addressed properly. There is thus a need to create awareness among adolescent girls so that they enjoy good health in the society.

REFERENCES

Blos, Peter, 1962, *On Adolescence: A Psychoanalytical Interpretation*. New York: Glencoe, Inc.

Census of India, 2001, *Registrar General and Census Commissioner 2001*. New Delhi: Government of India.

Centre for Development and Population Activities (CEDPA), 2001, *Adolescent Girls in India Choose a Better Future: An Impact Assessment*, available at www.cedpa.org/content/publications/detail/634 (accessed on 2 July 2007).

Cole, Leulla, 1962, *Psychology of Adolescence*, 5th ed. New York: Holt, Rinehart and Winston, p. 89.

Debold, Elizabeth, 1995, 'Helping Girls Survive the Middle Grades', *Principal*, 74(3): 22–4.

Ge, X., R.D. Conger and G.H. Elder Jr., 1996, 'Coming of Age Too Early: Pubertal Influences on Girls' Vulnerability to Psychological Distress', *Child Development*, 7: 3386–400.

George, A., 1994, 'It Happens to Us: Menstruation as Perceived by Poor Women in Bombay'. In *Listening to Women Talk about Their Health: Issues and Evidence from India*, edited by J. Gittelsohn, M.E. Bentley, P.J. Pelto, M. Nag, S. Pachauri, A.D. Harrison and L. Landman, New Delhi: Ford Foundation and Har Anand, pp. 168–83.

Indian Council of Medical Research (ICMR), 1992, *Task Force Study on Field Supplementation, Trial in Pregnant Women with 60 MG, 120 MG and 180 MG of Iron with 500 G of Folic Acid*. New Delhi: ICMR.

Patton, G.C., M.E. Hibbert, J. Carlin, Q. Shao, M. Rosier, J. Caust and G. Bowes, 1996, 'Menarche and Onset of Depression and Anxiety in Victoria, Australia', *Journal of Epidemiology and Community Health*, 50(6): 661–66.

Rice, F. Philip, 1990, *The Adolescent: Development, Relationships and Culture*, 6th ed. Boston, MA: Allyn and Bacon.

Shukla, S., 2005, 'Working on Menstruation with Girls in Mumbai, India. Vacha Women's Resource Centre', *EQUALS*, v(15): 4–5.

Tanner, J.M., 1972, 'Sequence, Tempo and Individual Variation in Growth and Development of Boys and Girls Aged 12 to 16'. In *Twelve to Sixteen: Early Adolescence*, edited by J. Kegan and Robert Coles, New York: W.W. Norton and Co.

Timothy, R. and S.I. Rajan, 2004, 'Awareness and Knowledge about HIV/AIDS in India: Evidences from RCH Survey (1998–99)', *Demography India*, 33(1): 61–83.

WHO, 2005, *Nutrition in Adolescence: Issues and Challenges for the Health Sector*. Issues in Adolescent Health and Development (WHO discussion papers on adolescence), WHO, available at http://www.who.int/child-adolescent-health/New_publications/ADH/WHO_FRH_ADH_ 97.9_en.pdf (accessed on 8 February 2007).

WHO, UNFPA and UNICEF, 1995, *Action for Adolescent Health*. Towards a Common Agenda, Recommendations from a Joint Study Group, available at http://www.who.int/child-adolescent-health/New_publications/ADH/WHO _FRH_ADH_ 97.9_en.pdf (accessed on 8 February 2007).

Wichstrom, L., 1999, 'The Emergence of Gender Difference in Depressed Mood During Adolescence: The Role of Intensified Gender Socialization', *Development Psychology*, 35: 232–45.

CHAPTER 10

Maternal Health among Rural Women: A Case Study in Dharwad District

Shakuntala C. Shettar

INTRODUCTION

There has been a perceptible change in recent years regarding the focus of development policies and priorities. In India, and globally, development goals are no longer defined in terms of economic growth exclusively. The vital link between health and development is increasingly recognized, and an attempt is made to reformulate health policies and programmes. Since women constitute nearly half of the total population in any society, their health status has implication for country's development and for a quality of life. The slogan *Healthy Women Healthy World* embodies the fact that as custodian of family health, women play a unique role in maintaining the health and well-being of their communities. Hence, the issue of women's health in general and reproductive health in particular came into prominence with the International Conference on Population and Development at Cairo in 1994 and the Fourth World Conference of women at Beijing in 1995. At these conferences, it was accepted that women's health and reproductive rights are important means of women's empowerment and quality of life.

The concept of women's health today has become a major concern in India because of high prevalence of infant, child, maternal mortality and deteriorating quality of life. Available evidences in India point to poor maternal and reproductive health status among women. Although India has made considerable progress in social and economic development, improvement in life expectancy, infant mortality and literacy rate, still it lagged behind in the improvement of women's health. India is one of the few countries where males significantly outnumber females (933 females for 1,000 males), and its maternal mortality rate in rural areas is among the world's highest. Women experience malnutrition, anaemia, infectious diseases and illness more than men and less likely to receive timely medical treatment. Women especially poor and rural women are often trapped in cycle of ill health exacerbated by childbearing and hard physical labour.

Therefore, the present paper is a modest effort in understanding maternal health in rural India so as to suggest some policy interventions for improving rural maternal health.

THEORETICAL FRAMEWORK

Maternal health refers to the health of women during pregnancy, childbirth and the postpartum period. It encompasses the health care dimensions of family planning, preconception, prenatal and postnatal care in order to reduce maternal morbidity and mortality. Preconception care can include education, health promotion, screening and other interventions among women of reproductive age to reduce risk factors that might affect future pregnancies. The goal of prenatal care is to detect any potential complications of pregnancy early, to prevent them if possible and to direct the woman towards appropriate specialist medical services as appropriate. Post-natal care issues include recovery from childbirth, concerns about newborn care, nutrition, breastfeeding and family planning. Maternal health problems also include complications from childbirth that do not result in death. For every woman who dies during childbirth, nearly 20 suffer from infection, injury or disability. Increasing contraceptive usage and family planning also improves maternal health through reduction in numbers of higher risk pregnancies.

Maternal mortality is an important indicator of maternal health. Most maternal deaths occur just before, during or just after delivery, often from complications that cannot be predicted and are difficult to prevent. Haemorrhage remains the leading cause of maternal death followed closely by sepsis, obstructed labour, hypertensive disorders of pregnancy and complications from unsafe abortion. Many times survival rates depend on the distance and time a woman must travel to get skilled emergency medical care. Delay in seeking care, in arriving at an emergency care facility and in receiving care from providers, raises mortality rates.

Poor maternal health is both an indicator and a cause of extreme poverty. According to Tamar Manuelyan Atnic, Vice President for Human Development World Bank 'Maternal deaths are both caused by poverty and are a cause of it. The costs of childbirth can quickly exhaust a family's income, bringing with it even more financial hardship.'

There are many socio-economic, cultural factors influencing maternal health and service utilization. And these factors operate at various levels—individual, household and community. In general, women in higher socio-economic groups tend to exhibit better maternal health and patterns of more frequent use of maternal health services than women in the lower socio-economic groups. Education of mother in particular is an important social variable that has a positive effect on the utilization of maternal and child health services. The other factors such as place of residence, religion and standard of living of the household are found to be important in the determination of the maternal health services. The poorer the household, the lack of access to skilled birth attendants during pregnancy and lower the educational attainment, the higher the risk of maternal death, which are preventable with increased political will and adequate financial investment.

LITERATURE REVIEW

Considerable researches have been done on women's health in India, which explain the leading determinants and causes of poor health in general, maternal health in particular. Many studies focus on the socio-economic, cultural factors that prevent women's access to health care services especially in rural areas.

Monica Sharma in her book *Women and Health: Problems and Issues* (1991: 197–215) has analysed different health issues of women as per 1981 census such as sex ratio, expectation of life, the age at marriage of women, nutritional status, childbearing practices, birth rate, abortions and so on. She summarized the situation regarding women's health as follows:

1. Inadequate basic health care facilities (including facilities of MCH, family planning, MTP and nutrition) for women and children in terms of outreach, range of services, quality and availability.

2. Major disparities in health care facilities to population groups in rural and urban areas: remote, backward, hilly and desert areas; and to socio-economically deprived groups.
3. Inefficient use of resources available for health care of women resulting in a slower pace of health development for them.
4. Poor health of women due to the synergistic effects of infection, malnutrition and uncontrolled fertility.
5. Ignorance and lack of knowledge related to health, nutrition and family planning affecting self-help efforts in health and resulting in under utilization of existing resources.
6. Social prejudices inherent in our milieu which affect the health of girls and women.
7. Absence or inadequacy of essential non-health facilities which affect health such as portable water, sanitation, female education and food supply.

C. Gopalan (1994) pointed out in his study that malnutrition among poor pregnant women in India is also widespread. Over 30 per cent of these women in the last stages of their pregnancy have been found suffering from severe anaemia.

K. Indira Bai et al. (1981) in a study conducted in an urban area of Tirupati and in rural area of Anantapur district found that 87.4 per cent of urban mothers know that mothers should take a good balanced diet where as in the rural areas only 58.12 per cent of mothers know this.

B.D. Bhatia et al. (1981) have studied 20 non-pregnant and non-lactating women from rural and urban areas of Varanasi to study the dietary intake. It was found that the mean daily intake of calories was inadequate in rural women.

Rafiqual Hund Chaudhury (1984) in his study indicates that the nutrient intake of pregnant women and lactating mother is far below that of others. Their consumption of calories and proteins relative to need is lower than that of non-pregnant and lactating women. Poor nutrition intake in developing countries is directly responsible for maternal deaths. A proper diet intake to a pregnant and lactating mother is very important.

Arora (2005) while explaining maternal mortality in Indian Scenario and its associated problems stressed the need for a strong and sustained government commitment, favourable policy of environment and well-targeted resources as a strategy for improving maternal health. She concluded that the existing health system does not adequately meet the needs of pregnant women, particularly for complications of pregnancy and obstetrical emergencies.

K. Navaneetham and A. Dharma Lingam (2000) in their paper 'Utilization of Maternal Health Care Services in South India' examined the patterns and determinants of maternal health care use across different social settings in South India: in the states of Andhra Pradesh, Karnataka and Tamil Nadu by using data from the National Family Health Survey (NFHS) carried out during 1992–93 across most states in India. The study focuses on most recent births to ever-married women that took place during the four years prior to the date of survey. They have used logistic regression models to estimate the effect of co-variates on the utilization of maternal health services, namely, antenatal care, tetanus toxoid vaccine, place of delivery and assistance during delivery. The study indicates that the determinants of maternal health care services are not the same across states and for different maternal health care indicators. Although illiterate women were less likely to use maternal health care services; there was no difference among the educated. The level of utilization of maternal health care services was found to be highest in Tamil Nadu, followed by Andhra Pradesh and Karnataka. Part of the interstate differences in utilization is likely to be due to differences in availability and accessibility among the three south Indian states. It is argued that the differential in access to health care facilities between rural–urban areas is an important factor for lower utilization of maternal health care services, particularly for institutional delivery and delivery assistance by health personnel in the rural areas of the three states. Results from this study indicate that health workers might play a pivotal role in providing antenatal care in the rural areas.

STATUS OF MATERNAL HEALTH

Global Scenario

Globally, every year over 500,000 women die of pregnancy-related causes, and 99 per cent of these occur in developing countries. More than 350,000 women die during pregnancy and childbirth every year. That is approximately 40 women every hour—34 per cent decline from the levels in 1990. Despite this decline, 99 per cent of maternal deaths occur in developing countries worldwide, the maternal mortality ratio (MMR) has decreased, with Southeast Asia seeing the most dramatic decrease of 59 per cent and Africa seeing a decline of 27 per cent. There are no regions that are on track to meet the Millennium Development Goal of decreasing maternal mortality by 75 per cent by the year 2015.

Although high-quality, accessible health care has made maternal death a rare event in developed countries, where only 1 per cent of maternal deaths occur, these complications can often be fatal in the developed world because the single most important intervention for safe motherhood is to make sure that a trained provider with midwifery skills is present at every birth, that transport is available to referral services and that quality emergency obstetric care is available. In 2008, 342,900 women died while pregnant or from childbirth worldwide. Although a high number, this was significant drop from 1980, when 526,300 women died from the same causes. This improvement was caused by lower pregnancy rates in some countries; higher income, which improves nutrition and access to health care; more education for women; and the increasing availability of 'skilled birth attendants'—people with training in basic and emergency obstetric care—to help women give birth. One specific disease that causes significant maternal health problems is HIV/AIDS. The transmission of HIV from mother to child in the developing world is a large concern; nearly 45 per cent of infected mothers transmit the disease to their children and HIV is a major cause of maternal mortality, leading to 60,000 maternal deaths in 2008. HIV rates are especially high in sub-Saharan and Eastern Africa, where maternal mortality rates are on the rise.

Almost 50 per cent of the births in developing countries still take place without a medically skilled attendant to aid the mother, and the ratio is even higher in South Asia. Women in sub-Saharan Africa mainly rely on traditional birth attendants (TBAs), who have little or no formal health care training. In recognition of their role, some countries and non-governmental organizations are making efforts to train TBAs in maternal health topics, in order to improve the chances for better health outcomes among mothers and babies.

Indian Scenario

India continues to contribute about a quarter of all global maternal deaths. Maternal health remains a significant problem in India. The important indicators of maternal health in India are age at marriage, maternal mortality, levels of fertility spacing between births, birth attendants, place of delivery, lack of access to health care and poor socio-economic status of women such as poverty, illiteracy, lack of autonomy, traditional beliefs and so on.

Each year in India, roughly 30 million women experience pregnancy and 27 million have a live birth. Of these, an estimated 136,000 maternal deaths and 1 million newborn deaths occur in each year and in addition, million more women and newborn suffer pregnancy and birth-related ill health. Rural women are among the most disadvantaged group in terms of maternal health. They are vulnerable to pregnancy risks and maternal deaths that are related to high levels of fertility, son preference, unsafe and lack of services, and lack of resources and knowledge. India had a high mortality ratio of nearly 407 deaths per 1 lakh births in 2004.

According to the available data nearly 20,000 deaths (about 18 per cent of all pregnancy- and child-related deaths) are related to unsafe deliveries and abortions of which most are occurring among the poor rural women. The National Family Health Survey (NFHS 2004–05) found that in the four years preceding the survey, 27 per cent of all pregnant women in India received no prenatal care during their pregnancies. Over 70 per cent of women attend at least one antenatal check-up, but only 37 per cent attend four or more times. Rural women are less likely to have a skill birth attendant present at their delivery. Only 47 per cent of women are delivered by a skilled attendant, and only 37 per cent of women have post natal care. World Health Organization estimates that 2.5 lakh health workers are required to ensure the delivery of essential healthcare to 80 per cent of the population. Studies have found that between 50 and 90 per cent of all pregnant women in India suffer from anaemia. Severe anaemia accounts for 20 per cent of all maternal deaths in India. Severe anaemia also increases the chance of dying from a haemorrhage during labour that accounts for 31 per cent of maternal deaths in India. With limited access to modern contraception and the lack of an enabling environment to use methods, women are impacted by too early, too frequent, too many pregnancies. The twin factors of distance to and cost of adequate care also increase chances of rural women dying as a result of pregnancy and childbirth complications. In addition, safe services are not available in India by rural women due to lack of resources and knowledge of the law. Many pregnant rural women cannot afford the costs associated with facility-based care, travel to reach a facility and do not receive adequate care. They are rarely exposed to comprehensive health information, about contraception, the importance of a skilled birth attendant, how to prevent HIV and a host of other important health issues. In the event of an obstetric emergency, delays in seeking help were increased by lack of transport, absence of decision makers, etc.

OBJECTIVES

The objectives of this paper are the following:

1. To understand the status of maternal health and consequent problems of rural women;
2. To analyse the socio-economic factors that interfere with their maternal health; and
3. To suggest measures in improving the maternal health of rural women.

METHODOLOGY

The data for this paper are based on the complete birth histories collected from the 200 ever-married women aged 20–49 years. The sample is selected from four villages of Kalaghatagi taluka, Dharwad district in Karnataka. They are Muttagi (50 samples), Herihonnihalli (100 samples), Sulikatti (25 samples), and Aralihonda (25 samples) according to the size of the eligible women population.

FINDINGS AND CONCLUSION

Socio-Economic Profile

As per Table 10.1, a majority of women respondents (53.50 per cent) were belonging to 24–29 age group. Nearly 29 per cent of them were illiterate and 46 per cent had completed only primary education. Seventy-nine per cent of them professed Hindu religion, and among them 47 per cent were belonging to Lingayat caste which is a dominant caste in this part of north Karnataka. Nearly 60 per cent of them were working as agricultural labourers, coolies, house workers and construction workers. A total of 74.5 per cent of them were having BPL card that indicates their poor economic standard. Fifty-four per cent of them even today are living in joint families.

Table 10.1 Socio-Economic Profile

Age Composition			*Literacy and Education*			*Religion*		
Age groups	*Number*	*%*	*Groups*	*Number*	*%*	*Religion*	*Number*	*%*
18–23	51	25.50	Illiterate	58	29.00	Hindu	158	79.00
24–29	107	53.50	Primary	92	46.00	Christian	1	0.50
30–35	34	17.00	High School	46	23.00	Muslim	32	16.00
36–41	8	4.00	PUC	4	2.00	Jain	9	4.50
Total	200	100.00	Total	200	100.00	Total	200	100.00
Type of Ration Card Holders			*Type of Family of Respondents*					
Ration card	*Number*	*%*	*Type of family*	*Number*	*%*			
APL	24	12.0	Joint	108	54.0			
BPL	149	74.5	Nuclear	92	46.0			
Anthodia	18	9.0	Total	200	100.0			
Other	9	04.5						
Total	200	100.0						

Maternal Health

The paper has analysed the following issues related to maternal health; they are birth attendants, place of delivery, number of children, spacing between births, still births and miscarriages, breast-feeding, family planning, medical check-up and health problems. The major findings are discussed further.

Birth Attendants and Place of Delivery

Table 10.2 shows that out of 200 respondents, 150 (80 per cent) respondents are delivered by a skilled attendant and 15 per cent from *dadis*, 2 per cent by midwife and remaining only 3 per cent by the senior member of a family.

It is evident from Table 10.3 that a great majority of respondents (i.e. 78 per cent) delivered in hospitals remaining 22 per cent, at home. Hence, the data indicate that although rural women are increasingly becoming aware of safe and hospital delivery, home deliveries are not totally ruled out from rural society. The primary health centres continue to provide major health facilities for rural women.

Table 10.2 Information about Birth Attendants

Birth Attendants	*Number*	*%*
Doctor	160	80.0
Nurse	29	14.5
Midwife	05	02.5
Senior member of a family	06	03.0
Total	200	100.0

Table 10.3 *Place of Delivery*

Place of Delivery	*Number*	*%*
House	46	21.9
Hospital	164	78.1
Total	200	100.0

Number of Children and Spacing between Births

Research on number of children and spacing between births indicate that the more the number of children, the greater the risk of maternal deaths, and the lesser the spacing between births, the more the risk for mother. Data in Table 10.4 clearly show that 54 per cent of women have three and more than three children, 25.5 per cent two and only 2 per cent have only one child.

Table 10.5 shows that 64.5 per cent of respondents are having children aged between one and five years, 26 per cent between 6–11 years and only 9.5 per cent have children above 12 years of age.

From Table 10.6, it is evident that 59 per cent of women reported spacing of two to three years between births and only 1 per cent having one-year difference. Hence, it is inferred that the idea of small family of two children is not yet ingrained among rural women and having more than three children is related to their desire of having at least one male child.

Table 10.4 Number of Children Desired by Respondents

Number of Children Desired	*Number*	*%*
One	5	2.5
Two	51	25.5
Three	109	54.5
More than three	35	17.5
Total	200	100.0

Table 10.5 Age of Children

Age of Children	*Number*	*%*
1–5 years	129	64.5
6–11 years	52	26.0
12–17 years	16	8.0
More than 18 years	3	1.5
Total	200	100.0

Table 10.6 Spacing between Births

Spacing between Births	*Number*	*%*
Up to 1 year	32	16.0
2–3 years	118	59.0
3–4 years	29	14.5
4–6 years	21	10.5
Total	200	100.0

Family Planning and Antenatal Check-Up

It is clear from Table 10.7 that 35 per cent of respondents have adopted tubectomy to control their births and 22 per cent have undergone laparoscopic operation. Not applicable respondents are those who are in the childbearing stage desirous of having one or two children. Vasectomy is totally not practiced among the respondents.

As evident from Table 10.8 that 88 per cent of women have undergone all general check-ups during their pregnancy such as blood pressure, blood check-up, urine and weight among them, 58 per cent have undergone antenatal check-ups for more than four times, 32 per cent two to four times and 8 per cent only once. This

Table 10.7 Family Planning Methods Adopted by Respondents

Family Planning Methods	*Number*	*%*
Mala-D	1	0.5
Copper-T incretion/IUCD	2	1.0
Tubectomy	70	35.0
Laparoscopic operation	44	22.0
Not applicable	83	41.5
Total	200	100.00

Table 10.8 *Respondents Go Through General Check-Ups During Their Pregnancy (BP, Blood Check-Up, Urine and Weight)*

Opinion	*Number*	*%*
Examined	196	98.0
Not examined	4	2.0
Total	200	100.0

Table 10.9 Complications during Childbirth

Complications	*Number*	*%*
Yes	22	11.0
No	178	89.0
Total	200	100.0

Table 10.10 *Number of Years Respondents Breastfeed Their Children*

Months/Years	*Number*	*%*
6 months	1	0.5
10 months	4	0.2
1 year	79	39.5
2–3 years	116	58.0
Total	200	100.0

shows that the idea of antenatal check-ups and taking care of their health during pregnancy is also emerging among rural women such as their counterparts in urban areas, which is a very welcoming trend in improving their maternal health.

As per Table 10.9, nearly 11 per cent of women reported complications during childbirth resulted in still births and miscarriages despite visiting hospitals and taking vaccination during pregnancy.

Table 10.10 shows the number of years respondents breastfed their children. Breastfeeding is generally considered good for children's health as that increases immunity. In general, mother should breastfeed for minimum one year. Accordingly, 58 per cent of women have breastfed their children for two to three years, 39.5 per cent of them for one year and only 2 per cent of them for 10 months.

Overall Health Status and Problems

Respondents were also asked to state their overall health status at present. Table 10.11 shows their present health status. Accordingly, 47.5 per cent of respondents report that their health is very good and they do not have any reproductive problems. Thirty-seven per cent said that though their health is good, on and often they suffer from some problems. Whereas 15.5 per cent said they are suffering from some health problems that are connected to their complications during pregnancy and childbirths.

Table 10.11 Respondents' Health Status

Health Status	*Number*	*%*
Good	95	47.5
Better	74	37.0
Somewhat good	31	15.5
Not good	00	00.0
Total	200	100.0

Table 10.12 *Information about Respondents' Health Problems during Last One Year*

Reasons for Ill Health	*Number*	*%*
Anaemia	5	2.5
Malnutrition	111	55.8
Anaemia, malnutrition, etc.	23	11.5
Anaemia, difficulty in delivery, etc.	6	3
Others	55	27.5
Total	200	100.0

As per Table 10.12, a majority of respondents (59.5 per cent) are suffering on and often from body and abdomen pains. They complained that these are the side effects of carelessness during their pregnancy and childbirths. As most of the women are anaemic, they often have problem of heavy bleeding, backache and body pain.

Knowledge about Blood Group

Table 10.13 reveals that a great majority of respondents (81 per cent) do not know their blood group. They said that though they

Table 10.13 Respondents' Awareness about Blood Group

Blood Group	*Number*	*%*
'A' positive	9	4.5
'B' positive	7	3.5
'AB' positive	12	6.0
'O' positive	9	4.5
'A' negative	1	0.5
Do not know	162	81.0
Total	200	100.0

had undergone blood check-ups during their pregnancy they are not aware of their blood group.

SUGGESTIONS

The present study is a modest effort in revealing certain facts about women's maternal health in rural India. It is evident from the study that rural women are increasingly becoming aware of safe delivery, which is a positive trend in improving maternal health. They are taking care about their health during pregnancy and undergoing antenatal check-ups as their counterparts in urban areas. Although, family planning adoption has been universal among rural women, vasectomy is a remote possibility. Primary Health Centres continue to play an important role in providing maternal health services to rural women. Despite this, they are subjected to many health problems resulting from complications during pregnancy and childbirth and suffering from easily curable health problems such as anaemia and malnutrition. The idea of institutional delivery and skilled birth attendant is not totally entrenched among rural women due to their illiteracy and poverty.

Hence, the maternal health in rural India can be improved by making concerted efforts along with the following lines:

1. Rural women must be informed well about the existing health facilities to protect from maternal risks through mass media, health workers and so on.
2. The role of primary health centres, auxiliary nurse midwives must be increased to create awareness among rural women.
3. Regular health check-ups, blood check-up camps should be made through Anganwadi and other health workers.
4. Since the maternal risks are related to lack of infrastructure facilities, bad roads, care should be taken to tackle these problems by the government.
5. The role of 108 ambulances should be increased and extended to rural areas.
6. Health education of couples to make them understand the importance of antenatal check-ups, hospital deliveries and small family norms.
7. Initiative from the government would be of paramount importance in this effort. This would include allocation of sufficient funds to all the health institutions including primary health

centres. Even more important is to ensure that the funds actually reach the users.

8. Widespread availability of medicines and other iron tablets to the remotest areas.
9. Accountability in case of the unfortunate event of any maternal death. Taking appropriate remedial measures for preventing lapses noted in the management of these cases will be of immense value in reducing the maternal mortality.

CONCLUSION

The existing health system does not adequately meet the needs of pregnant women, particularly for complications of pregnancy. Three major problems need to be addressed: (1) widespread illiteracy among the rural women; (2) shortage of standard medicines and trained staffs at referral facilities; and (3) a lack of knowledge of emergency transport. National government, non-government organizations and social workers must commit to addressing policy barriers to improve maternal health, including efforts to increasing resources for health care systems.

REFERENCES

Arora, Punita, 2005, 'Maternal Mortality: Indian Scenario', *MJAF*, 61(3): 214–15.

Bhatia, B.D., D. Banerjee, D.K. Agarwal and K.N. Agarwal, 1981, ' "Dietary Intakes of Urban and Rural Pregnant Lactating and Non Pregnant", Non-Lactating Vegetarian Women in Varanasi', *Indian Journal of Medical Research*, 74: 680–87.

Chaudhury, Rafiqual, 1982–84, *Social Aspect of Fertility with Special Reference to Developing Countries*. New Delhi: Vikas Publishing House.

Gopalan, C., 1994, 'Some Aspects of Nutrition in India'. In *Population in India's Development 1947–2000*, edited by Ashish Bose, A. Mitra, P. Desai and J. Sharma, New Delhi: Vikas Publishing House, pp. 101–08.

Indira Bai, K., V.N. Sastry and C.C. Obula Reddy, 1981, 'A Comparative Study of Feeding Pattern of Infants in Rural and Urban Areas', *The Indian Journal of Paediatrics*, 49: 277–80.

Navaneetham, K. and A. Dharma Lingam, 2000, *Utilization of Maternal Health Care Services in South India*. Trivandrum:

Seshadri, Subadra, 2008, 'Nutritional Anaemia in South Asia'. In *Malnutrition in South Asia: A Regional Profile*, edited by Stuart Gillespie, Kathmandu: Regional Office for South Asia, UNICEF.

Sharma, Monica, 1991, 'Women and Health: Problems and Issues'. In *Sociology of Health in India*, edited by T.M. Dak, Jaipur: Rawat Publications, pp. 196–216.

Wikipedia, free encyclopedia.en.wikipedia.org/wiki/Maternal-health

www.womendeliver.org/knowledge-centre facts...maternal-health

www.unicef.org/india/health.

CHAPTER 11

Child and Maternal Health in Uttar Pradesh: A Study on the Impact of ASHA

Nida Siddiqui

Good health is a prerequisite for human welfare and development. A healthy community forms the infrastructure upon which an economically viable society can be built. Good health confers on a person or on groups, freedom from illness and the ability to realize one's potential. Good health and long life are valued attainments in themselves. It provides the opportunity to develop abilities and use one's innate potential in pursuit of personal goals. Being healthy and being able to live long also brings some indirect benefits of individual to the society as a whole.

The common indicators of health status are life expectancy at birth, infant mortality rate, fertility rate, crude birth rate and crude death rate. These indicators of health are determined by numerous factors such as per capita income, nutrition, housing, sanitation, safe drinking water, social infrastructure, health and medical care services provided by government, geographical climate, employment status, incidence of poverty and the like.[1]

The level of health and health problems varies from one country to another, one region to another. There are developed countries such as the United States, the United Kingdom, etc. where people suffer from entirely different health problems ranging from increased use of technology to obesity in contrast to a developing country such as India where a 'common' man can only think of such 'high society diseases'. Even within India, there is a huge contrast, where, on the one hand, a vast majority of people are struggling hard to make both ends meet, whereas on the other hand, there is prodigious food waste in Indian weddings, which clearly depicts the intra-regional difference.

The current health situation in India is a sad story of deprivation, unless one is fobbed off by the display of hi-tech medical care and the use of state-of-the-art medical technologies in five star deluxe facilities of a few selected urban centres; however, the tale of utter helplessness and callous carelessness is so apparent that it is now frequently taken as a matter of course. The blatantly paradoxical spectacle of buying and selling of health improvements as consumer goods by the well-off minority in the metros on the one hand and the denial of basic health facilities to the vast majority of the rural population along the length and breadth of the country on the other hand hardly evokes any comment.

The access to healthy living condition and good quality health care is not only the basic human rights for all citizens but also essential prerequisites for socio-economic development. However, the inequality in social, economical or political context between various population groups in the Indian society has a direct bearing on its health indicators. Millions of people in developing countries are trapped in poverty, malnutrition, hunger and disease, although there are regional variations in living conditions, but the most vulnerable among them are the rural section of the society who have very limited access to resources. The resources are generally short; the World Health Organization (WHO) has identified a global deficit of nearly 4.3 million health workers.[2] The use of para-professional health workers has been implemented in several countries to close the health worker gap. While community health workers cannot replace a weak health system, they can perform valuable tasks such as case management for common illnesses, promotion of health behaviour, immunization and community.[3]

In India, the latest band of community-based functionaries, named accredited social health activist (ASHA), were proposed under the National Rural Health Mission (NRHM) who serve the population of 1,000 in hilly areas and 500 in desert terrain in rural areas. ASHA is the first port of call for any health-related demands of deprived sections of the population, especially women, children, old aged, sick and disabled people. She is the link between the community and the health care provider.[4] The focus of the present paper is to find out the impact of ASHA on maternal as well as child health in Aligarh district of Uttar Pradesh (UP).

OBJECTIVES OF THE STUDY

1. To analyse the health conditions in general and maternal and child health in particular in the state of UP
2. To study the impact of ASHA on the child and maternal health

METHODOLOGY

Study Area

The study was undertaken in Aligarh District of Uttar Pradesh State. There are a total of 12 blocks and 859 villages in Aligarh District. Total population of Aligarh is 2,992,286, with 1,607,402 males and 1,384,884 females.[5]

Sampling

The study area had a total of 2,200 ASHAs who were selected under the NRHM. Following the census method, the data were collected from 150 ASHAs in Jawan block of Aligarh district.

Data Collection and Tools

An interview schedule was used for data collection, which comprised of both closed as well as open-ended questions. To further support the study, a 360-degree appraisal method was used in which focused group discussions (FGDs) were held with ASHAs, community members and mother-in-laws of the community members.

Variables

The independent variables were divided into ages of 20–25 years, 25–30 years, 30–35 years, 35–40 years, 40–45 years and above 45 years; highest level of education was divided into illiterate, up to 8th, 10th, 12th graduation and above. The dependent variables were scored on the diet of pregnant women as advised by ASHA (excellent, very good, good, average and poor), health check-ups advised by ASHA during pregnancy (four, three, two, one, do not know), household visit made by the ASHA (once, once in every 15 days, once a week, twice a week, thrice a week, more than thrice), and finally the first visit made by ASHA after the delivery (within 1 hour, within 24 hour, within first week, within first 14 days). Finally, data were cleaned and entered into SPSS version 16 software for analysis. Cross tables and frequency tables have been made with the help of the software.

HEALTH STATUS OF INDIA AND UTTAR PRADESH

India carries a large burden of the world's disease, as one would expect given its large population and high levels of poverty. It is estimated that acute forms of protein energy malnutrition affects 35 per cent of school children in Africa, 16 per cent in Asia and 4 per cent in Latin America. Similarly, it is estimated that two-thirds of pregnant women in the developing country would suffer from nutritional anaemia. High maternal and infant mortality rates are closely linked with inadequate maternal and child care services.[6]

There is no unique 'Indian' health status but rather a diversity of state-level situations. Health conditions in Kerala are comparable to those in the upper-middle-income countries such as Trinidad, Argentina and Mauritius. Most Indian states, however, are comparable to lower-middle-income countries such as Brazil, Egypt and Peru. Conditions in the poorest-performing states are similar to those in low-income countries such as Sudan, Nigeria and Tanzania.[7] If one compares India's health burden with that of the world, one can easily notice the large burden of world's disease on India's health burden mainly due to its large population and high levels of poverty. India has a major portion of the world's child and maternal deaths as well as a disproportionate amount of the disease burden due to tuberculosis, leprosy and immunizable diseases.[8] In comparison with its share of the world population, India has high levels of deaths due to traditional childhood infectious diseases such as acute lower respiratory infections (pneumonia), diarrhoea, measles and tetanus.[9]

When one talks about the health scenario at the national level, India's life expectancy has shown remarkable improvement, rising from 49 years in 1970 to 63 years in 1998. Similarly, infant mortality dropped from 146 deaths per thousand births in the 1950s to 70 in 1999 and to 58 in 2005,[10] while the total rate fell significantly from 6.0 in the 1960s to 3.3 in 1999[11] to 2.9 in 2005. Although Indians no longer suffer from the waves of famine that marked earlier periods in the nation's history, recent survey has shown that the infant mortality in UP stood at 72 deaths per 1,000 births as compared to the all-India average of 58.[12]

There has been progress on several health development parameters such as the overall decline in childhood mortality, maternal mortality and incidence of preventable diseases in UP, but this is far below satisfactory in comparison to other states and developing countries. For instance, over the past decade (1990–2001), while Bangladesh and Nepal recorded a progress of 46 per cent and 37 per cent, respectively, in reduction in child mortality, India's progress was 24 per cent and UP showed lower performance than the national average.[13] Uttar Pradesh is lagging behind from many states in terms of health indicators such as life expectancy, infant mortality, etc. Nearly 71 per thousand of children in UP die before reaching the age of one year.[14]

Deaths during the neo-natal period (within 28 days of life) contribute to almost 64 per cent of the infant mortality in the state. As per the National Family Health Survey-II (NFHS-II), UP had the highest Under 5 Mortality Rate in the country (122.5 deaths per 1,000 live births as compared to the all-India average of 94.9).[15]

The latest survey of NFHS-III (2005–06) shows that only 23 per cent of children (12–23 months) were found to be fully immunized against the six vaccine preventable diseases. Findings of NFHS-III reveal that although the state's total fertility rate is high (3.8), there is a dismally low prevalence of antenatal care (ANC) and birth-related counselling being provided to pregnant women in the state. As per the survey, only 26 per cent of the pregnant women in the state received three or more ANCs. The share of institutional deliveries in the state stands at only 22 per cent. The nutritional status of women is also poor. Almost 50 per cent of women in the state suffer from some form of anaemia. In 1997, there were an estimated 707 maternal deaths per 100,000 live births (Sample Registration Survey 1997), almost 70 per cent higher than the national average of 437, as per the recent Sample Registration Survey (2001–03), the maternal mortality stands at 517 per 100,000 live births while the national average is that of 301.[16]

UP's achievement on major health indicators is ranked among the lowest in India (see Table 11.1). In the past five years, only one-quarter of pregnant women made three or more ANC visits for their last birth, and nearly three of four deliveries took place at home. The interplay among the large unmet need for family planning (33.8 per cent), six relatively low literacy levels, high levels of rural

Table 11.1 Key Health Indicators

Seven Indicators	*Uttar Pradesh*	*India*
Crude Birth Rate SRS 2007	29.5	23.1
Crude Death Rate SRS 2007	8.5	7.4
Total Fertility Rate SRS 2007	3.9	2.7
Infant Mortality Rate SRS 2007	69	55
Maternal Mortality Ratio SRS 2007	440	254
Female Literacy Rate (Census, 2001) (%)	42.2	53.7

poverty and gender disparities results in poor maternal health and extraordinarily high maternal mortality ratios, infant mortality rates and fertility rates.[17]

NUTRITIONAL PROFILE OF UTTAR PRADESH

Uttar Pradesh, in particular, has very high levels of malnutrition despite large stocks of food grains resulting from increased agricultural productivity. Nutritional indicators of the state are one of the poorest in the country with large interregional imbalances. High levels of malnutrition particularly among women and children have been directly and indirectly influencing mortality rates in infants, children and women. NFHS-III data indicate that out of 10 children under three years, almost five are underweight and four are stunted. High incidence of general under-nutrition and micronutrient deficiency is reflected in the high childhood mortality and infant mortality.

Uttar Pradesh is lagging behind in health indicators such as life expectancy, infant mortality rate, etc. Nearly, 71 per thousand of children in UP die before reaching the age of one.[18] The fate of the mother is also not very happening, every year 38,000 women die in the state while delivering a child. Almost half of the deaths occur at home and another 10 per cent to 15 per cent mothers die on the way to the hospital.[19] On an average, 80 per cent of pregnant women are anaemic. Actually, mothers' health depend on a number of factors, right from conception the health of the child is directly linked with that of the mothers' health, but it is quite sad to note that in UP only about half of the total pregnant women get ANC services.[20] Malnutrition among mothers is high. It is estimated that 80 per cent of women marry and give birth before the age of 18 years. Maternal mortality rate in UP is eight times higher than in Kerala and 70 per cent higher than the national average.

India's 72 million children are malnourished, and UP accounts for 10–12 million of these malnourished children. It is alarming to note that UP has 52 per cent prevalence of under-nutrition, with every second child below three years of age suffering from chronic undernutrition. Malnutrition among children is one of the biggest public health problems in UP. It adversely affects the growth and development of children, including their learning ability, and the capacity to cope with the problems of daily living. Every sixth undernourished child in India lives in UP and every second child in UP is undernourished. It is a sad reminder that UP ranks fourth with respect to prevalence of underweight children in India.[21]

INITIATIVES TAKEN

At the time of India's independence, health care services in India were scant, predominantly urban, hospital based and curative. The National Family Planning Programme was launched in 1952 with emphasis on population control. The maternal and child health (MCH) programme has evolved over a period of time.

Evolution of Maternal and Child Health Programmes in India

From time to time, various programmes for the improvement in maternal and child health have evolved in our country starting from Family Planning Programme, 1952, adopted by the Government of India (GoI), which was followed by the Department of Family Planning, 1961, created in the Ministry of Health, then 1971 Medical Termination of Pregnancy (MTP) Act 1971, then in 1977 renaming Family Planning to Family Welfare followed by 1978 Expanded Programme on Immunization (EPI), then in 1985 Universal Immunization Programme (UIP) + National Oral Rehydration Therapy (ORT) Programme, then in 1992 Child Survival and Safe Motherhood Programme (CSSM), which was followed by 1996 Target-Free Approach; 1997 Reproductive and Child Health

Programme-1 (RCH-1), and finally 2005 Reproductive and Child Health Programme-2 (RCH-2).

Practices to Improve Maternal, Newborn and Child Health

The major goal of the Department of Family Welfare is to reduce maternal mortality and morbidity. Several new initiatives have been taken in this regard. The focus has undergone a paradigm shift from individualized vertical interventions to a more holistic and integrated life-cycle approach, giving more focused attention to the reproductive health care and more recently to give greater emphasis to child health, while other changes and innovations were being implemented to improve maternal, newborn and child health include:[22]

1. Training of MBBS doctors in anaesthetic skills for emergency obstetric care at First Referral Units (FRUs).
2. Setting up of blood storage centres at FRUs.
3. Development of guidelines for skilled attendance at birth for auxiliary nurse midwives/lady health visitors (ANMs/LHVs) and guidelines for normal pregnancy and management of obstetric complications, including authorizing ANMs/LHVs to be able to conduct a limited number of identified lifesaving midwifery skills and practices.
4. Guidelines for operationalizing FRUs and 24-hour delivery services at Primary Health Centre (PHCs).
5. Universalization of Integrated Child Development Services (ICDS)—There is a proposal in Union Budget 2005–2006 to create 188,168 additional Anganwadi centres to attain universalization of ICDS as per existing population norm. The allocation for ICDS has been increased from Rs 1,623 million in 2004–2005 to Rs 3,142 million for the year 2005–2006.
6. Janani Suraksha Yojna (National Maternity Benefit Scheme) is envisaged as a package of services, geared at reducing maternal mortality, neonatal mortality, female feticide and gender disparity.
7. In the new initiative, NRHM, every village/large habitat will have a female ASHA chosen by and accountable to the *panchayat* to act as the interface between the community and the public healthcare system.

ASHA—A Ray of Hope

Most countries have largely relied on females as Community Health Workers (CHWs).[23,24] Although both men and women are employed at grass-roots level, there is a collective impression (particularly amongst policy makers) that female workers are able to deliver care more effectively than male workers at community level.

Global experience shows that women, even when briefly trained, can successfully increase the coverage of health care, particularly if they are locally recruited and made accountable to the local clients (Global Equity Initiative, 2004). The introduction of the ASHA is thus an important and welcome step.[25] Simultaneously, there has been found to have an inverse relationship between the density of health workers and maternal mortality, infant and child mortality, and vaccination prevalence.[26,27]

In 2004, Dr. N.H. Antia, the eminent social health activist and a pioneer in community health worker programmes led a team of civil society representatives to the Prime Minister's Office to present a note on the concerns on the narrow definition of the ASHA. This intervention contributed to the creation by the Ministry of Health and Family Welfare (MoHFW), of a multi-stakeholder task force to design the ASHA programme, and this led to the official definition of the roles and responsibilities of the ASHA.[28]

The accredited social health activist is called by the acronym ASHA, which in Hindi means 'hope'. She must be a primary resident of the village with formal education up to the eighth class, and preferably in the age group of 25–45 years. She is selected by the *Gram Sabha* through an intense community mobilization process, and is provided with training. She is also equipped with a drug kit. After selection, ASHA is given induction training for 23 days spread over a period of 12 months. ASHA is also given periodic training, re-training and on-the-job training. She acts as a mobilizer, facilitator and a link between ANM at sub-centre, *Anganwadi* worker (under the Integrated Child Development Services programme) and the community, and play a major role in forging ownership of the community for the health programme.[29]

ROLES AND RESPONSIBILITIES OF ASHA

ASHA is the first port of call for any health-related demands of deprived sections of the population, especially women and children, who find it difficult to access health services. She has to ensure better access to universal immunization, safe delivery, newborn care, and prevention of water-borne and other communicable diseases, nutrition and sanitation. She is accountable to the *panchayat*, and is entitled to receive performance-based compensation for providing health services. Presently, ASHA is working at the lowest hierarchical level in primary health care. ASHA will be a health activist in the community who will create awareness on health and its social determinants and mobilize the community towards local health planning and increased utilization and accountability of the existing health services. She would be a promoter of good health practices. She will also provide a minimum package of curative care as appropriate and feasible for that level and make timely referrals. Her roles and responsibilities would be as follows[30]:

ASHA will take steps to create awareness and provide information to the community on determinants of health such as nutrition, basic sanitation and hygienic practices, healthy living and working conditions, information on existing health services and the need for timely utilization of health and family welfare services. She will counsel women on birth preparedness, importance of safe delivery, breastfeeding and complementary feeding, immunization, contraception and prevention of common infections including reproductive tract infections/sexually transmitted infections (RTIs/STIs) and care of the young child. ASHA will mobilize the community and facilitate them in accessing health and health-related services available at the village/sub-centre/primary health centres, such as immunization, antenatal check-up, antenatal care (ANC), post-natal check-up (PNC), ICDS, sanitation and other services being provided by the government. She will work with the Village Health and Sanitation Committee of the Gram Panchayat to develop a comprehensive village health plan.

She will arrange, escort/accompany pregnant women and children requiring treatment/admission to the nearest pre-identified health facility, that is, Primary Health Centre/Community Health Centre/First Referral Unit (PHC/CHC/FRU). ASHA will provide primary medical care for minor ailments such as diarrhoea, fevers and first aid for minor injuries. She will be a provider of directly observed treatment, short-course (DOTS) under Revised National Tuberculosis Control Programme. She will also act as a depot holder for essential provisions being made available to every habitation such as oral rehydration therapy (ORS), iron folic acid tablet (IFA), chloroquine, disposable delivery kits (DDKs), oral pills and condoms, etc. A drug kit will be provided to each ASHA. Contents of the kit will be based on the recommendations of the expert/technical advisory group set up by the Government of India. Her role as a provider can be enhanced subsequently. States can explore the possibility of graded training to her for providing newborn care and management of a range of common ailments particularly childhood illnesses. She will inform about the births and deaths in her village and any unusual health problems/disease outbreaks in the community to the sub-centres/Primary Health Centre. She will promote construction of household toilets under Total Sanitation Campaign. Fulfilment of all these roles by ASHA is envisaged through continuous training and up gradation of her skills, spread over two years or more.

RESULTS

A total of 150 ASHAs were interviewed for the study. The present study was conducted in Jawan block of Aligarh district; majority of the ASHAs were selected in the year 2006. Their ages ranged from 20 to above 45 years, although the maximum age for selection of ASHA is 45 years, but it was found out that 16 ASHAs were above 45 years, as they have been working since 2006 at an age quite close to 45 years, and since then their service has not been terminated. The majority were between 40 and 45 years (30 per cent) followed by the age group 30–35 years (25.3 per cent). The 25–30 age group contributed 16 per cent and 35–40 were 13.3 per cent, whereas 20–25 age group made up only 4.7 per cent and 10.7 per cent of the ASHAs were above 45 years. A total of 87.3 per cent of ASHAs were married, 11.3 per cent were widowed and only 1.3 per cent was separated. About 93.3 per cent of the ASHAs were Hindus, 6 per cent were Muslims and only seven per cent belonged to Jain community. A total of 60.7 per cent of the ASHAs were that of upper caste, whereas 39.3 per cent belonged to lower caste.

A good many, that is, 59.3 per cent of the ASHA's husbands' monthly income was up to Rs 3,000, followed by 25.3 per cent whose husbands' income was in the range of Rs 3,000–6,000, which is further followed by 4.5 per cent having husbands' monthly income in the range of Rs 6,000–9,000 and only seven per cent belonging to the category where husbands' monthly income was in the range of Rs 9,000–12,000.

With regard to the level of education, 48 per cent of ASHAs were educated up till 8th class, 28 per cent had completed 10th class, 12.7 per cent had attained education till 12th class, 4.7 per cent had achieved tertiary education and above, whereas 6.7 per cent of ASHAs did not have any formal education at all.

In selection of ASHAs, ANMs have played an important role as 36 per cent of the total ASHAs were selected by ANMs, followed by 30.7 per cent who were selected by village *panchayat*, 16.7 per cent were selected by entire village, 12.7 per cent by other leader and only 4 per cent by health officers.

As per the guidelines given under NRHM Gram Sabha meeting must be held while selecting ASHA, it was found out that 44 per cent of the ASHAs had a gram sabha meeting during their selection, whereas 54.3 per cent reported that there was no gram sabha meeting during their selection, and only a small number, that is, 7 per cent were unaware about the selection procedure. Only 7.3 per cent of ASHAs were involved in any other community-based voluntary work before joining as an ASHA, whereas 92.3 per cent were not involved in any such community-based voluntary work.

Tables 11.2 and 11.3 discuss the relationship between the variables measured and tested while collecting the data.

EFFECT OF EDUCATION ON HEALTH OF MOTHER AND CHILD

In Table 11.2, excellent diet refers to a diet consisting of green leafy vegetables, non-vegetarian, milk/milk products, gur and fruits; very good diet refers to milk, gur, fruits and vegetables; good diet refers to vegetables, milk and fruits; and average diet consists of milk/milk products and green vegetables, whereas poor diet refers to green leafy vegetables only. ASHAs must be educated up till 8th class as per the guidelines given by the government. From Table 11.2, it is quite clear that the higher the level of education, the better the diet recommended by the ASHAs; however, one must also notice that the level of education cannot be the sole criteria to determine the performance of ASHA, as not even a single illiterate ASHA recommended poor diet to the pregnant women, whereas the ASHAs who are educated up till 10th and 12th classes have recommended poor diet.

Table 11.2 Education of ASHA and her Performance

Education Level of ASHA							*Total*
		Illiterate	Up to 8th	Up to 10th	Up to 12th	Graduation and above	
Diet of pregnant women as advised by ASHA							
	Excellent	0	9	3	3	2	17
	Very good	1	18	14	5	2	40
	Good	5	36	18	9	2	70
	Average	4	7	6	0	1	18
	Poor	0	2	1	2	0	5
	Total	10	72	42	19	7	150
Health check-ups advised by ASHA during pregnancy							
	Four	1	8	4	0	1	14
	Three	5	39	22	11	6	83
	Two	1	19	11	7	0	38
	One	2	5	3	1	0	11
	Do not know	1	1	2	0	0	4
	Total	10	72	42	19	7	150

(Continued)

Table 11.2 (Continued)

Education Level of ASHA							*Total*
		Illiterate	Up to 8th	Up to 10th	Up to 12th	Graduation and above	
Household visit by ASHA							
	Once in every 15 days	2	2	2	0	0	6
	Once a week	3	6	11	3	1	24
	Twice a week	3	36	21	12	5	77
	Thrice a week	2	25	6	3	1	37
	More than three times	0	3	2	1	0	6
	Total	10	72	42	19	7	150
First visit, made by ASHA after the delivery	Within 1 hour	2	9	5	2	0	18
	Within 24 hour	5	54	33	16	7	115
	Within first week	2	8	4	1	0	15
	Within first 14 days	1	1	0	0	0	2
	Total	10	72	42	19	7	150

Studies have shown that CHWs with higher educational qualifications have opportunities for alternative employment and therefore migrate from one job to another, and therefore do not deliver good services to the community,[31] as it was found out while doing FGDs with ASHA, that ASHAs with higher education were searching for other services, and the major reason for joining here was incentives as one of them said with much pride

> *humne toh BA kari hai hum toh ANM bhi ban saktin hain, pati ne kaha tha ki izzat ki naukri hai char paise bhi kama legi kar le isliye kar li, ab jahan zyada paise milenge wahin naukri karenge* (I have done BA and can be considered for the post of ANM also, my husband told me that this is a reputed job where i can earn some money so i have joined it, but now I will do job where I will earn more money.)

While conducting the interview, it was found out that out of the five illiterate ASHAs, three of them had recommended the use of *kadhai* (iron pan) for making food as it helps in raising the iron content of vegetables, hence it can be said that although the level of education can be a determining factor, it is the level of awareness, knowledge and dedication towards the work which can actually affect the performance of an ASHA.

It was observed that there exists a positive relation between the level of education and the advice given for health check-ups. The higher the education level, the higher was the number of health check-ups advised by the ASHAs. But it was observed that 50 per cent of the ASHAs who said they do not know about the health check-ups were educated till 10th class, whereas 55.3 per cent of the total ASHAs irrespective of their education level recommended at least three health check-ups.

Further, it was found out that although education does have some impact on household visits, there is no such direct relationship. ASHAs comprising 51.3 per cent of the total, irrespective of their education level, visited household in the community twice a week, moreover there is one thing in common in the ASHAs who were illiterate as well as whose education level was higher than graduation, that is, ASHAs in both the groups on the extreme end did not visit more than thrice in a week.

It was also found out that there is a positive relationship between the level of education and the first visit made by the ASHA. Moreover, it should also be noted that 76.7 per cent of ASHAs have visited the baby during the first hour, which is a very positive step in saving the precious lives. First visit is an important factor in determining the infant mortality rate, as during the first hour of birth of baby, the colostrum is released from the mother's milk, which has numerous health benefits and long life span for both mother and baby. The fact is also supported by a study on the association between the use and knowledge of colostrum on neonatal and post-natal deaths occurred in Varanasi, which found that the neonatal and post-natal deaths were very low for females who were familiar with the importance of colostrum and feeding it.[32]

EFFECT OF AGE ON HEALTH OF MOTHER AND CHILD

Although no clear trend can be noticed between age and diet of pregnant women advised by ASHAs from the above Table 11.2, it can be noticed that the ASHAs in the age group of 20–25 years do not recommend poor and average diet, which shows that ASHAs in this age group are more aware as they themselves are in their active reproductive period, and therefore can understand all the requirements of a woman easily. Only 15.3 per cent of ASHA recommend average and poor diet which itself is a very clear indication about the good performance of ASHA.

It was observed that 51.3 per cent of the ASHAs have visited household twice a week. As the age increases, there is increase in the household visit by the ASHAs.

It was further established that 55.3 per cent of ASHAs have advised the pregnant mothers to take at least three check-ups during pregnancy of which blood test, urine test and abdominal examination were known by a majority of them, whereas few of them also knew about the weight test. On being interviewed, the ASHAs generally said *teen jaache karati hain hum* (there are three check-ups advised by us); sometimes, it was hard for them to name the respective check-ups, but all they knew was that they had to take a pregnant mother for three check-ups. Again it should be noted that the health check-ups advised by ASHAs increases as the age increases and more specifically in the age group of 35–40. While the advice of ASHAs in the age group on the two extreme ends, that is, 20–25 and > 45 was almost the same.

Table 11.3 Age of ASHA and her Performance

Age of ASHA		*20–25*	*25–30*	*30–35*	*35–40*	*40–45*	*> 45*	*Total*
Diet of pregnant women as advised by ASHA	Excellent	1	4	2	3	3	4	17
	Very good	1	4	10	8	14	3	40
	Good	5	11	21	7	21	5	70
	Average	0	4	3	2	6	3	18
	Poor	0	1	2	0	1	1	5
	Total	7	24	38	20	45	16	150
Household visit by ASHA	Once in every 15 days	0	1	3	1	1	0	6
	Once a week	1	4	9	1	6	3	24
	Twice a week	4	9	21	13	24	6	77
	Thrice a week	2	9	5	3	12	6	37
	More than three times	0	1	0	2	2	1	6
	Total	7	24	38	20	45	16	150

(Continued)

Table 11.3 (Continued)

Age of ASHA								*Total*
		20–25	*25–30*	*30–35*	*35–40*	*40–45*	*> 45*	
Health check-ups advised by ASHA during pregnancy								
	Four	1	3	1	4	2	3	14
	Three	2	13	23	12	24	9	83
	Two	3	4	8	4	15	4	38
	One	1	3	4	0	3	0	11
	Do not know	0	1	2	0	1	0	4
	Total	7	24	38	20	45	16	150
First visit made by ASHA after the delivery								
	Within 1 hour	0	3	6	5	4	0	18
	Within 24 hour	6	19	27	14	35	14	115
	Within first week	1	2	5	1	4	2	15
	Within first 14 days	0	0	0	0	2	0	2
	Total	7	24	38	20	45	16	150

Although no clear-cut relationship between the age and first visit after the delivery can be determined, it was noted that 76.7 per cent of the ASHAs have visited within the first 24 hours of the delivery of the child, ASHAs in the age group of 35–40 are the best performers. While the ASHAs in the age group on the two extreme ends, that is, 20–25 and > 45 did not make any visit in the first hour of the birth of the child.

While conducting the interview, it was also found out that 100 per cent of the ASHAs have advised the mother to give the first milk to the child, 100 per cent of them have counselled mothers to breastfeed exclusively and 100 per cent of ASHAs have also educated women about complimentary feeding, which should be done only after six months. A majority (96 per cent) of ASHAs have advised the mother to keep the baby warm and dry.

All of them have reported that during the initial years of their work, they faced resistance from the community and were not accepted, especially resistance was faced while changing the habit of colostrums feeding as a general trend was found in both Muslims as well as Hindus, that they discard the first milk of the mother because they consider it impure.

According to an ASHA, Muslim people discard the colostrums as they say they will give mother's milk only after seeing the moon, whereas the Hindus in general earlier considered it to be impure, and they give the milk only after the *chhathi* (the sixth day after the birth of the child when name is given to the baby generally by the paternal aunt of the child) of the child and they discard mother's milk on the earth as they think it will help in protecting the child from evil spirits.

To further support the study focussed group discussions were conducted with grandmothers as well as the community members. It was found out that although the ASHA were advising the mother on taking good health care of the child; however, still there are certain lacunas present in our society which need to be dealt in an efficient manner. While conducting interview, it was found out that 100 per cent of the ASHAs were advising mothers to give colostrums to the child, but through FGDs it was found out there is still a strong prevalence of the old tradition to give ghutti/water/honey/buffalo milk/pehuwa (a local food made from jaggery and ajwain, which is considered good in order to clean the stomach of the infant) instead of colostrums. It was also found out that although the mother was informed by the ASHAs about the importance of the first milk, but they are restricted by the elder members of their family especially their mothers-in-law play an important role in carrying such old traditions.

Again contradictions in actual performance was found out while discussing the issue of exclusive breastfeeding up till six months in FGDs as it was reported by some of the grandmothers that they do not allow their daughters-in-law for exclusive feeding as it will deteriorate the health of the child, and it is necessary according to them to give additional diet in the form of buffalo's milk/cow milk and water in the first six months of the birth of the baby.

While discussing the issue of keeping the child warm and dry, it was found that although mother considered it to be essential to keep the baby warm but their ways were varying from wrapping the child in warm clothes, to application of hot oil on the umbilicus of the child. A few of them were also adopting the method of Kangaroo Mother Care (KMC) to keep the baby warm.

Talking about the diet advised by ASHA, it was found out during FGDs with community members that although they were advised good diet and they knew the concept of square meal (a colourful meal) consisting of colours namely white (egg/milk/fish/rice), yellow (pulses/fats/fruits), green (green leafy vegetables), red (orange/fruits/meat/chicken), but very few actually take good diet as their general response was *jee nhn karta hai zyada khane ka mitli aati hai jab bachcha hota hai andar, us samay aur dino se bhi kam khaya jaata hai* (don't feel like eating during pregnancy, there is a nausea feeling and even one eat less in comparison to other days).

CONCLUSION

It is beyond any doubt that the wealth of a country is judged by the health of its people. Admittance of healthy living conditions and good quality health is not only fundamental right for each and every Indian but also crucial factor for socio-economic maturity of the nation. Especially the status of health in rural India may be one of the worst in the world where women carry tremendous burden of work, hence there was an urgent need to have some torch bearers in the society. The above study tries to explore out the impact of education level and age of ASHA on maternal and child health, who were launched under NRHM in 2005 as a 'change agent' to bring out the reforms in improving the health status of oppressed community of India.

This study aimed at establishing how selected socio-demographic characteristics of ASHA affected the health of the mother as well as child. Results showed that age of ASHA, level of education of the ASHA affected the diet of pregnant women advised by ASHA, household visits by ASHA, health check-ups advised by ASHA during pregnancy, first visit after the delivery by ASHA.

A higher education level was related to better performance in all parameters except household visit made by ASHA. This result concurs with a study in Nigeria (Ande, 2004) which observed that literate CHWs could learn and enhance skills and therefore deliver services better.[33] It was also found out that even ASHAs who were less educated were performing at par with the ASHAs who were higher in education. However on further analysis, it was also noticed that ASHAs who were educated up till 8th class to 12th class were found to be the best performers.

Age was found to have a positive effect on household visits made by ASHA and advice given by ASHA on health check-up visits, while no such relationship was observed on recommendation of diet by ASHA and first visit after delivery by ASHA. The age group 35–40 years appeared to be the most appropriate for selection of community health workers in order to obtain optimum results. Younger and much older ASHAs had sub-optimal performance. This differs from a study in Uganda (Kallander et al., 2006), which found that factors such as age, sex and education had no effect on the CHWs performance.[34]

The health scenario has undergone change with the efforts of the government at regular intervals but as one knows that, it is the rural section which is the most deprived and the needy one, and for this ASHAs are working at the lowest hierarchical level. From the above study, it can be said that although ASHAs are imparting knowledge and working in the community, still much needs to be done to get results on implementation level, as certain lacunas in the form of old-age tradition, practices, careless behaviour among the respondents towards their health is still prevailing, which was found out through FGDs, which is a long way to go and can only be done through regular visits and more and more counselling as change is not a rapid action, rather it comes slowly with time.

NOTES

1. R.V. Dadibhavi and S.T. Bagalkoti, 'Inter-State Disparities in Health Status in India', *Yojana*, Vol. 38, No. 23, 1994, pp. 17–21.
2. J.J. Hall and R. Taylor, 'Health for All Beyond 2000: The Demise of the Alma Ata Declaration and Primary Health Care in Developing Countries', *Medical Journal of Australia*, Vol. 178, 2003, pp. 17–20.
3. A. Haines et al., 'Achieving Child Survival Goals: Potential Contribution of Community Health Workers', *Lancet*, Vol. 369, 2007, pp. 2121–31.
4. Womens' Empowerment in NRHM: A Case Study of ASHA (Accredited Social Health Activist), available at http://www.ssmrae.com/admin/images/602d5d794d4dd1e279272d7c1a04b5e8.pdf (accessed on 16 November 2011).
5. www.censusindia.gov.in/Census_Data_2001/Village_Directory/View_data/Village_Profile.aspx (accessed on 28 October 2011).
6. C.P. Yadav, *Empowerment of Women*, vol. 1. Lucknow & New Delhi: Laxmi Shikshan Sansthan and Anmol Publications Pvt. Ltd., 2000, p. 47.
7. David H. Peters et al., published for the World Bank by Hindustan Publishing Corporation (India) Better Health Systems for India's poor, Findings, analysis, and options, 2002, p. 267.
8. Ibid, p. 269.
9. Ibid, p. 270.
10. 2005, Sample Registration System, April, Ministry of Home Affairs, New Delhi.
11. 2000, Sample Registration System Bulletin, April. Ministry of Home Affairs, New Delhi.
12. 2004, Sample Registration System Bulletin, April. Ministry of Home Affairs, New Delhi.
13. Human Development Report, Uttar Pradesh.
14. Ibid.
15. Indian Institute for Population Science, 2000, (NFHS-2) 1998–99, Bombay: IIPS.
16. Indian Institute for Population Studies & Macro International, 2007 NFHS (NFHS-3) 2005–06, India, Vol. 1, Mumbai: IIPS.
17. Prevention of Mother to Child Transmission of HIV: An RCH–HIV Integration Model for Uttar Pradesh, available at http://www.

healthpolicyinitiative.com/Publications/Documents/1340_1_PMTCT_RCH_HIV_Integration_India_UP_FINAL_acc.pdf (accessed on 26 July 2012).

18. Human Development Report, Uttar Pradesh, 2007.
19. Ibid.
20. Ibid.
21. Ibid.
22. Improving Maternal, Newborn and Child Health in the South-East Asia Region, available at www.searo.who.int/linkfiles/Improving_maternal_newborn_and_child_health_india (accessed on 3 August 2012).
23. D.E. Bender and K. Pitkin, 1987, 'Bridging the Gap: The Village Health Worker as the Cornerstone of the Primary Health Care Model', *Social Science & Medicine*, Vol. 24, No. 6, pp. 515–28.
24. U. Lehmann, I. Friedman and D. Sanders, 2004, 'Review of the Utilization and Effectiveness of Community-Based Health Workers in Africa', *JLI Working Paper 4–1: Human Resources for Health and Development*.
25. Health of the National Rural Health Mission, available at www.indiaenvironmentportal.org.in/files/NRHM (accessed on 16 November 2011).
26. WHO, *WHO Estimates of Health Personnel: Physicians, Nurses, Midwives, Dentists, Pharmacists*. Geneva, Switzerland: World Health Organization, 2000.
27. L. Chen et al., 'Human Resources for Health: Overcoming the Crisis', *Lancet*, Vol. 364, 2004, pp. 1984–90.
28. ASHA Which Way Forward Executive Summary—Evaluation of ASHA Programme, available at http://nhsrcindia.org/download.php?downloadname=pdf_files/resources_thematic/Community_Participation/NHSRC_Contribution/ASHA_Which_way_forward_-_Evalaution_of_ASHA_Programme_Report_NHSRC_417.pdf (accessed on 18 December 2013).
29. Human Resources for Health in India's National Rural Health Mission: Dimension and Challenges, available at www.searo.who.int/linkfiles/Regional_Health_Forum_Volume_10_No_1_03Human_Resources_for_Health_in_Indias_National (accessed on 16 November 2011).
30. Guidelines on Accredited Social Health Activist (ASHA), available at http://mohfw.nic.in/NRHM/RCH/guidelines/ASHA_guidelines.pdf (accessed on 5 February 2012).
31. A. Brown et al., 'On the Front Line of Primary Health Care: The Profile of Community Health Workers in Rural Quechua Communities in Peru', *Human Resources for Health*, Vol. 4, 2006, p. 11.

32. K. Singh and P. Srivastava, 'The Effect of Colostrum on Infant Mortality: Urban Rural Differentials', *Health and Population: Perspectives and Issues*, July-December 1992, pp. 153–54; 94–100.
33. O. Ande, O. Oladepo and W.R. Brieger, 'Comparison of Knowledge on Diarrhoeal Disease Management between Two Types of Community Based Distributors in Oyo State Nigeria', *Health Education and Research*, Vol. 19, No. 1, pp. 110–13.
34. Ndedda Crispin et al., 'Effects of Selected Socio-Demographic Characteristics of Community Health Workers on Performance of Home Visits during Pregnancy: A Cross-Sectional Study in Busia District', *Kenya Global Journal of Health Science*, Vol. 4, No. 5, 2012, p. 84.

REFERENCES

Ande, O., O. Oladepo and W.R. Brieger, 2004, 'Comparison of Knowledge on Diarrhoeal Disease Management between Two Types of Community Based Distributors in Oyo State Nigeria', *Health Education and Research*, 19(1): 110–13.

Bender, D.E. and K. Pitkin, 1987, 'Bridging the Gap: The Village Health Worker as the Cornerstone of the Primary Health Care Model', *Social Science & Medicine*, 24(6): 515–28.

Brown, A., R. Malca, A. Zumaran and J.J. Miranda, 2006, 'On the Front Line of Primary Health Care: The Profile of Community Health Workers in Rural Quechua Communities in Peru', *Human Resources for Health*, 4: 11.

Chen, L., T. Evans, S. Anand, J.I. Boufford, H. Brown, M. Chowdhury, M. Cueto, L. Dare, G. Dussault, G. Elzinga, E. Fee, D. Habte, P. Hanvoravongchai, M. Jacobs, C. Kurowski, S. Michael, A. Pablos-Mendez, N. Sewankambo, G. Solimano, B. Stilwell, A. de Waal and S. Wibulpolprasert, 2004, 'Human Resources for Health: Overcoming the Crisis', *Lancet*, 364: 1984–90.

Crispin, Ndedda, Annah Wamae, Meshack Ndirangu, David Wamalwa, Gilbert Wangalwa, Patrick Watako and Elijah Mbiti, 2012, 'Effects of Selected Socio-Demographic Characteristics of Community Health Workers on Performance of Home Visits During Pregnancy: A Cross-Sectional Study in Busia District', *Kenya Global Journal of Health Science*, 4(5): 84.

Dadibhavi, R.V. and S.T. Bagalkoti, 1994, 'Inter-State Disparities in Health Status in India', *Yojana*, 38(23): 17–21.

Global Equity Initiative, 2004, *Joint Learning Initiative; Harvard University Global Equity Initiative*. Cambridge, MA: Global Equity Initiative: Distributed by Harvard University Press.

Haines, A., D. Sanders, U. Lehmann, A.K. Rowe, J.E. Lawn, S. Jan, D.G. Walker and Z. Bhutta, 2007, 'Achieving Child Survival Goals: Potential Contribution of Community Health Workers', *Lancet*, 369: 2121–31.

Hall, J.J. and R. Taylor, 2003, 'Health for All Beyond 2000: The Demise of the Alma Ata Declaration and Primary Health Care in Developing Countries', *Medical Journal of Australia*, 178: 17–20.

Kallander, K., G. Tomson, X. Nsabagasani, J.N. Sabiiti, G. Pariyo and S. Peterson, 2006, 'Can Community Health Workers and Caretakers Recognize Pneumonia'. In *Scaling up Health and Education Workers: Community Health Workers*, edited by F. Abbatt, London: DFID Health Systems Resource Centre.

Lehmann, U., I. Friedman and D. Sanders, 2004, 'Review of the Utilization and Effectiveness of Community-Based Health Workers in Africa', *JLI Working Paper 4–1: Human Resources for Health and Development*.

Singh, K. and P. Srivastava, 1992, 'The Effect of Colostrum on Infant Mortality: Urban Rural Differentials', *Health and Population: Perspectives and Issues*, July-December: 153–54; 94–100.

WHO, 2000, *WHO Estimates of Health Personnel: Physicians, Nurses, Midwives, Dentists, Pharmacists*. Geneva, Switzerland: World Health Organization.

Yadav, C.P., 2000, *Empowerment of Women*, vol. 1. Lucknow & New Delhi: Laxmi Shikshan Sansthan and Anmol Publications Pvt. Ltd., p. 47.

CHAPTER 12

Antenatal Care and Delivery of Health Practices among the Muslim Women of Yangbi Village of Imphal East, Manipur

Rajiya Shahani

Antenatal care (ANC) is the systemic medical supervision of women during pregnancy. It aims at preserving the physiological aspect of pregnancy and labour and to prevent or detect, as early as possible, all that are pathological. World Health Organization defines ANC as a dichotomous variable, having or had one or more visits to a trained person during the pregnancy. It includes a routine follow-up provided to all pregnant women at primary care level from screening to intensive life support during pregnancy and up to delivery. Early diagnosis during pregnancy can prevent maternal ill health, injury, maternal mortality, foetal death, infant mortality and morbidity. Hence, the earlier a pregnant woman comes under the supervision of an obstetrician, the better will be the maternal care.

Several studies during the past few decades have identified three key elements to reduce maternal mortality and improve neonatal health, that is, family planning, skilled birth attendance for all deliveries and access to emergency obstetric care for all women with life-threatening complications (Freeman et al., 2007). Maternal care includes care during pregnancy and should begin from the early stages of pregnancy. According to a survey report of IIPS 1995, 100,000 women in India are estimated to die every year from pregnancy- and childbirth-related causes re-enforces the importance of ensuring that all pregnant women receive adequate ANC during pregnancy, and the deliveries take place under the supervision of trained medical personnel in a hygienic environment. Women can access ANC services either by a health centre where such services are available or from health workers during their domiciliary visits. The former gives an idea about the voluntary utilization of the institutions, whereas the latter is related to the quality aspect of the service. One of the most important components of ANC is to offer information and advice to women about pregnancy-related complications and possible curative measures for early detection and management of complications.

ANC can also play a critical role in preparing a woman and her family for birth by establishing confidence between the woman and her health care provider and by individualizing promotional health messages (WHO, 1996). Further, antenatal visits may raise awareness about the need for care during delivery or give women and their families a familiarity with health facilities that enable them to seek help more efficiently during a crisis (Sai and Measham, 1992; Mondal, 1997). However, uptake of these services is far from universal even in settings where they are widely available. While ANC is considered essential for the health of both the mother and the child, it is important to analyse the possible factors contributing to its utilization. The Indian Council of Medical Research (ICMR) has been engaged in studies focusing on developing strategies for improving maternal and child health (MCH) and family planning (FP) services at grass root levels for over a decade. With a shift in focus from MCH and FP towards comprehensive reproductive health care, the ICMR initiated a project on Integrated Reproductive Health Care Delivery through its network of Human Reproduction Research Centres (HRRCs) located at medical colleges in various regions of the country.

The proposed paper aims at studying ANC of mother with an implication for the childbirth and child development. It is mainly based on primary data of 100 women selected through simple random sampling and collected with the help of interview schedule.

The study is conducted to examine the relationships between ANC measures and socio-economic variables among the Muslim women of Yangbi Khunou, a village of Imphal East, Manipur. The village they belong to is about 10–12 km from the main city of Manipur (Imphal), and around five to six kilometres from the Imphal East district headquarter (Porompat). This small village lies near the Nongmaiching mountain range and surrounded by paddy fields from all the directions. The village has a total population of around 541 persons, who reside in a total of 91 houses. The total population comprises 248 male populations and 298 female populations. They live in kachcha houses with unhygienic and unsanitary toiletry systems. They do not have access to improved source of drinking water. On an average, the education level of the study area counts to be almost a nil as they are found to have attended the schools or any other educational institutions up to junior level of class fifth/sixth or less. This village has a lower primary school and no primary health centre or sub-centre; the nearest primary health centre is about three kilometres away. In short, the basic socio-economic condition of the study area is very poor; so that they are deprived well to absorb to the mainstream of basic amenities.

The study was conducted among the married Muslim women of Yangbi Khunou Village in Imphal East district, Manipur. A hundred married women in the 15 to 49 year-old age group were chosen for the study and it has been conducted through interview schedule; simultaneously, group discussion and informal interview method. Observation has been made through semi-participants method. Interview schedule were prepared centrally in English and were translated into regional language (Manipuri). The questions pertaining to women's perceptions, opinions, knowledge, attitudes, etc. were open-ended.

BACKGROUND PROFILE OF MANIPURI WOMEN'S REPRODUCTIVE HEALTH

According to the DLHS-3 2007–08, the information on basic indicators of reproductive health services, provided that currently married women aged 15–44 years had full antenatal check-ups for about 12.5 per cent only. The situation was even worst in rural areas, where they altogether accounted for only about 9.1 per cent as against 27.5 per cent in urban areas. The complete information regarding such indicators is provided in Table 12.1, which further shows that the total institutional delivery stood at 41.1 per cent that was only 38.6 per cent for rural areas. In most of the cases, delivery of child happened to be at home, which accounted for 58.2 per cent for the state and 65.5 per cent for the rural areas. Safe delivery stood for only about 55.8 per cent. Moreover, although the women folk in this category heard or knew about the HIV/AIDS (95.7 per cent), they had little knowledge about the reproductive tract infections/ sexually transmitted infections (RTIs/STIs) (20 per cent). In another case, the information about the unmarried women aged 15–24 years showed that they considered (89 per cent) family life education or sex education important; however, only about half of them (40.2 per cent) received it. The women in this age group were well aware of contraception of various kinds. Like the case of married women, the unmarried women in this age group also had little knowledge about the RTIs/STIs.

Table 12.1 Some Basic Indicators of Women Reproductive Health of Manipur

Indicator	*Total* (%)	*Rural* (%)	*Urban* (%)
Indicators based on currently married women (aged 15–44 years)			
Antenatal Care			
Mothers who received any antenatal check-up	75.4	71.4	92.9
Mothers who had antenatal check-up in first trimester	57.3	51.2	84.4
Mothers who had three or more ANCs	57.5	50.8	87.2
Mothers who had at least one tetanus toxoid injection	73.8	69.7	91.9
Mothers who consumed 100 IFA tablets	37.9	38.6	35.0
Mothers who had full antenatal check-ups	12.5	9.1	27.5
Delivery Care			
Institutional delivery	41.1	33.8	73.6
Delivery at home	58.2	65.5	25.8
Delivery at home conducted by skilled health personnel	14.7	14.3	16.7
Safe delivery	55.8	48.3	90.3
Mothers who received post-natal care within two weeks of delivery	42.9	35.4	76.2
Mothers who received financial assistance for delivery under Janani Suraksha Yojana or JSY	6.3	5.7	9.1
Awareness of RTI/STI and HIV/AIDS			
Women who have heard of RTI/STI	47.7	42.5	70.8
Women who have heard of HIV/AIDS	95.7	94.8	99.5
Women who have any symptoms of RTI/STI	20.0	21.3	14.2

(Continued)

Table 11.3 (Continued)

Women who know the place to go for testing of HIV/AIDS	56.7	51.9	76.6
Women who underwent test for detecting HIV/AIDS	19.9	16.5	34.1
Other Reproductive Health Problems			
Women who had primary or secondary infertility	7.3	7.3	7.2
Women who had problem of obstetric fistula	1.4	1.5	0.8
Indicators based on unmarried women (aged 15–24 years)			
Family Life Education			
Unmarried women who opined family life education/sex education important	89.0	88.5	91.3
Unmarried women who ever received family life education/sex education	40.2	38.1	49.7
Awareness of Contraceptive Methods			
Unmarried women who knew about condom	93.9	93.4	96.3
Unmarried women who knew about pills	82.1	80.4	90.0
Unmarried women who knew about emergency contraceptive pills or ECPs	20.3	18.2	30.6
Unmarried women who ever discussed about contraception with anyone	20.4	18.5	29.5
Awareness of RTI/STI and HIV/AIDS			
Unmarried women who have heard of RTI/STI	41.7	37.9	59.7
Unmarried women who have heard of HIV/AIDS	97.7	97.4	98.8
Unmarried women who knew the place for testing of HIV/AIDS	54.2	52.1	64.0
Unmarried women who underwent test for detecting HIV/AIDS	0.9	0.9	0.7

Source: DLHS-3 (2007–08).

The observations related to ANC and delivery health practices among Muslim women of Yangbi Khunou are as follows.

DEMOGRAPHIC CHARACTERISTICS OF THE STUDY POPULATION

Socio-economic conditions greatly affect the health status, either negatively or positively. It is therefore, important to consider the role of social, cultural, health system and economic factors that impact on maternal health, and ultimately maternal mortality. A woman's decision to seek health care could be affected by the influence of her partner or other family members; social norms; her education; her status in society; the distance she lives from the clinic; how sick she is; her previous experiences with the health system and how she expects to be treated by health care providers; her level of decision-making power in the household; and her access to credit, land and income (Lule et al., 2005). According to Garro (1998), there are four key criteria relevant for treatment choice: (1) gravidity of the illness, (2) whether an appropriate home remedy is known for the illness, (3) faith or confidence in the effectiveness of home remedies for a given illness and (4) expense of treatment and the availability of resources.

Table 12.2 Demographic Characteristics of the Study Population

Variable	*No. of Samples*	*Percentage*
Respondents' Age Group		
Less than 16	10	10
16–25	30	30
26–35	40	40
36–45	15	15
More than 45	5	5
Respondents' Occupation		
Farmer	30	30
House-wife	60	60
Others	10	10
Respondents' Education Level		
None	60	60
Primary	35	35
Secondary	5	5
Post-secondary	0	0
Education Level of Respondents' Husbands		
None	10	10
Primary	50	50
Secondary	30	30
Post-secondary	10	10

Table 12.2 shows the basic demographic characteristics of the study population. It is confirmed from the table that the socio-economic conditions of the population studied is not sound. Despite, majority of the women aged between 16 and 35 years, most of them are housewives and a few of them engage in agricultural activities. They hardly attended the educational institutions beyond primary level, but their husbands attended beyond secondary level.

BASIC ANTENATAL CHECK-UPS

ANC refers to pregnancy-related health care provided by a doctor or a health worker in a medical facility or at home. Generally, ANC visits after confirmation of pregnancy should be scheduled at intervals of four weeks thereafter (MacDonald and Pritchard, 1980). However, women from low socio-economic groups and others are advised for the ANC visits in a minimum at regular intervals for once, twice, thrice and fourth (Park and Park, 1989). Pandey et al. (2004) in their study found that the neonatal mortality is lower among children whose mothers received three or more ANC check-ups as compared to those children born to mothers who either did not receive ANC check-up or received less than three check-ups. The utilization of maternal health care services, however, varies from society to society and within society from individual to individual. It depends on a large number of socio-economic–cultural–demographic–psychological factors, which operate at community and individual levels (Das, 2000).

It can be found from the Table 12.3 that shows the antenatal check-ups by the mothers, around 50 per cent of the mothers neither acquired any medical facility at primary health centre or sub-centre, or at any other hospital or maternity home nor at home. Some do only for once. There is negligence of antenatal care, and unawareness and negative attitudes regarding the availing of health care services.

ANC includes the provision of iron and folic acid tablets, tetanus immunization and others. This provision prevents various complications at different stages of the pregnancy. For instance, iron deficiency anaemia among mothers is a major threat to safe motherhood and to health and survival of infant because it contributes to low birth weight, lower resistance to infection and impaired development (Pandey et al., 2004).

Table 12.3 Antenatal Check-Up by the Mothers

Antenatal Check-Up(s)	*No. of Samples*	*Percentage*
Once	35	35
Twice	10	10
Thrice	5	5
Never	55	55

Table 12.4 Medical Aids during Antenatal Care

Medical Aids Availed	*No. of Samples*	*Percentage*
Tetanus immunization	20	20
Iron and folic acid tablets	10	10
Did not avail any medical aids	70	70

From Table 12.4, it can be noted that nearly one-third of mothers in the population under study do not take any such tablets or injections. A few mothers go only for tetanus immunization. On the other hand, they also do not take experts' advice on appropriate diets.

Even when women are aware of the importance of a nourishing diet during pregnancy, socio-economic constraints deny them access to better nutrition (Khan et al., 1988). Table 12.5 provides the common food items that are usually taken by the mothers during

Table 12.5 Food Items

Food Items	*No. of Samples*	*Percentage*
During Pregnancy		
Vegetables	80	80
Fruits	10	10
Milk	5	5
Meat	5	5
After Delivery		
Plain rice with dried fish	60	60
Plain rice with boiled vegetable	30	30
Honey	5	5
Milk	5	5

their pregnancy and after child delivery. Mostly, they go for the normal food items during pregnancy and plain rice with dried fish or boiled vegetables.

DELIVERY OF CHILD

Safe motherhood and health and survival of the child are the most preferable choices of all the mothers and their families. It is advised to seek assistance from trained/skilled personnel at the time of delivery. Skilled attendant refers to people with midwifery skills (including doctors, midwives and nurses) who have been trained to proficiency in the skills necessary to manage normal deliveries and recognize, diagnose, manage or refer obstetric complications (UNFPA, 2004). It also includes advice on referral to institutional delivery in case of complication, along with regular medical care.

As there is neither any health worker nor primary health centre or sub-centre, or any private maternity home, most of cases favoured to choose traditional *Dai* (Maibie) for about 55 per cent, while comparatively few prefer for doctors (around 30 per cent). This can be provided by Table 12.6 that shows the types of attendants at the time of delivery and place of delivery. Moreover, unable to afford the cost for the institutional deliveries and others, most of the deliveries take place at homes. These are the two general principles that enable us to understand their choice: (1) for non-severe illnesses, actions are cost-oriented. People start with less-costly treatments (home treatment) and only opt for more costly alternatives if the first treatments

Table 12.6 Attendants at the Time of and Place of Delivery

Response	*No. of Samples*	*Percentage*
Attendants		
Dai	5	5
Doctor	35	35
Traditional Dai (maibie)	55	55
Health worker	10	10
Place		
Hospital	30	30
Primary Health Centre	Nil	Nil
Home	70	70

Table 12.7 Cutting and Dressing the Naval Cord

Cutting Instrument Used	*No. of Samples*	*Percentage*
New blade	80	80
Scissor	15	15
Others	5	5

Dressing Material Used	*No. of Samples*	*Percentage*
Dettol	55	55
Powder	5	5
Cloth	40	40

fail or if they do not know the treatment for the problem; (2) for illnesses considered serious, illness costs are secondary, and treatment selection primarily depends on 'probability of cure', and normally persons opt for a physician (Garro, 1998).

Since majority of the deliveries takes place at homes with traditional *Dais,* instruments/devices and other medicinal materials employed should be considered for the hygienic and some other purposes. Three out of four women deliver at home, usually in unhygienic conditions, and two out of three continue to be delivered by untrained attendants (including *Dais*) (IIPS, 1995). In a familiar case, as shown in Table 12.7, health problems to the mothers during last delivery, blades (used in shaving razors) are used for cutting the naval cord; and for dressing, instead of medicated cotton and bandages, pieces of cloth with some antiseptics such as Dettol are used. Desirable aseptic precautions were not always taken when cutting the cord, as they do not appear to use sterile cord care kits. Such practices are risky and will obviously result in excessive bleeding, infection, etc.

With a number of socio-economic and health-related infrastructural constraints and negligence of health care during antenatal period, the mothers are found to be reported for certain health problems. Table 12.8 shows the common health problems faced by the mothers during their last baby delivery. Common ones include body weakness in around 40 per cent of the mothers and excessive bleeding in about 30 per cent.

Table 12.8 Health Problems to the Mothers during Last Delivery

Health Problems	*No. of Samples*	*Percentage*
Swelling	10	10
Excessive bleeding	30	30
Weakness	40	40
Immense pain	10	10
Not faced any problem	10	10

Table 12.9 Medical Aid during Complications or Health Problems at Delivery

Response	*No. of Samples*	*Percentage*
Communicated maibies	25	25
Communicated doctors	60	60
Not faced any problem	15	15

Numerous factors contribute to poor access to health care, delay in identifying and reaching medical facilities and delay in receiving adequate and appropriate treatment (Thadeus and Maine, 1994). These factors lead women to face a number of problems related to their health as well as their babies' health. Although, complications are reported, a few of them sought treatment only when the symptoms were severe. This contributes to encountering certain complications at the time of delivery. Table 12.9 shows medical aid during complications or health problems at the time of delivery. Only in such cases have the mothers consulted doctors in general. Very often, they used to communicate with traditional *Dais* (maibies) too.

In general, most of the pregnant women are advised to take maximum rest and exercise on a regular basis. Even after delivery, they are required to take some rest and avoid working hard. Table 12.10

Table 12.10 Work Done during Pregnancy

Types of Work	*No. of Samples*	*Percentage*
Fetching water from rivulet and pond	35	35
Working in the fields	20	20
Household work	40	40
Others	5	5

Table 12.11 Span of Taking Rest after Delivery

Span of Taking Rest (Days)	*No. of Samples*	*Percentage*
5–10	55	55
10–15	20	20
15–20	15	15
20–25	10	10

lists down the types of work done during pregnancy. Unfortunately, not a single mother takes rest before delivery; they used to do routine works of their daily life such as fetching water from the rivulet and pond, working in the fields, and doing other household works.

Moreover, regarding the span of taking rest after delivery, it is found that maximum women take 5–10 days' rest after delivery. The information related to this is given in Table 12.11—span of taking rest after delivery. Most of the mothers take rest for about 5–10 days (55 per cent) and 10–15 days (20 per cent).

On the basis of the findings and discussion, the study reveals that the unawareness among the Muslim women of Yangbi Khunou Village is the major factor, which deprives them from using the proper ANC and scientific health care practices. The mothers who do not seek the proper ANC practices are mostly uneducated. Apart from illiteracy and unawareness, there are some other factors that act as barriers in adopting modern practices of antenatal health; some of these are distant from the health services centre, deemed unnecessary; inconvenience to accept or avail facilities; no botheration shown by the husbands, elders and health staff; etc.

The finding suggest the need to inform about the availability of benefits to ANC and modern delivery health care services to help them overcome the traditional attitude and other hurdles that prevent them from seeking ANC and delivery health practices. The literacy of women as well as husbands is the key to improve ANC of pregnant women. Hence, effort should be made to have information, education and communication (IEC) activities targeted to educate the mothers, specially, in rural areas and there should be focus on the national RCH programmes. That is, the gap that presently exists between the health care needs of adolescent girls and RCH programme must be formulated in a new method of delivery of health services considering the social, cultural, economical and political contexts.

REFERENCES

Das, M., 2000, 'Reproductive Health Issues and Health Seeking Behaviour of Women in a Matrilineal Set-up: A Study of Khasi Tribal Women', Ph.D. Thesis, International Institute for Population Sciences, Mumbai.

Freeman, L.P., W.J. Graham, E. Brazier, J.M. Smith, T. Ensor, V. Fauveau, E. Themmen, S. Currie and K. Agarwal, 2007, 'Practical Lessons from Global Safe Motherhood Initiatives: Time for a New Focus on Implementation', *Lancet*, 370(9595): 1383–91.

Garro, L., 1998, 'On the Rationality of Decision-Making Studies: Part 1: Decision Models of Treatment Choice', *Medical Anthropology Quarterly*, 12(3): 319–40.

IIPS, 1995, *National Family Health Survey (MCH and Family Planning), 1992–93*. Mumbai: International Institute for Population Sciences.

Khan, M.E., R. Anker, G. Dastidar and S. Bairathi, 1988, 'Inequalities between Men and Women in Nutrition and Family Welfare Services: An In-depth Enquiry in an Indian Village', *Social Action*, 38(4): 398–417.

Lule, E., G.N.V. Ramana, N. Oomman, J. Epp, D. Huntington and J.E. Rosen, 2005, 'Achieving the Millennium Development Goal of Improving Maternal Health: Determinants, Interventions and Challenges', *Health, Nutrition and Population (HNP) Discussion Paper*, The World Bank, Washington, DC.

MacDonald, P.C. and J.A. Pritchard, 1980, *Williams Obstetrics*, 16th ed. New York: Appleton-Century-Crofts.

Mondal, S.K., 1997, 'Utilization of Antenatal Care Services in Rajasthan', *Family Welfare Journal*, 43: 28–33.

Pandey, A., B.N. Bhattacharya, D. Sahu and R. Sultana, 2004, 'Are Too Early, Too Quickly and Too Many Births are High Risk? An Analysis of Infant Mortality in India Using National Family Health Survey', *Demography India*, 33(2): 127–57.

Park, J.E. and K. Park, 1989, *Textbook of Preventive and Social Medicine*, 12th ed. Jabalpur: Banarsidas Bhanot Publishers.

Sai, F.T. and D.M. Measham, 1992, 'Safe Motherhood Initiative: Getting Our Priorities Straight', *Lancet*, 339: 478–80.

Thadeus, S. and D. Maine, 1994, 'Too Far To Walk: Maternal Mortality in Context', *Social Science in Medicine*, 38(8): 1091–110.

UNFPA and the University of Aberdeen, 2004, *Maternal Mortality Update 2004: Delivering into Good Hands*. New York: UNFPA.

World Health Organization (WHO), 1996, *Care in Normal Birth: A Practical Guide*. Geneva: WHO/FRH/MSH 96–24.

CHAPTER 13

Role of Maternal Locus of Control in Infant and Young Child-Feeding Intervention in Rural India

Sylvia Fernandez Rao, N. Balakrishna, Patrice L. Engle, Margaret (Peggy) Bentley and Shahnaz Vazir

INTRODUCTION

Infant and young child-feeding (IYCF) interventions often focus on knowledge improvement of caregivers to facilitate behaviour change. While nutrition education intervention to improve infant and young child feeding have been successful (Guldan et al., 2000; Bhandari et al., 2004) literature also shows caregiver characteristics such as intelligence, education and nutritional status play a role in improving child growth and development (Aruna et al., 2001; Wachs et al., 2005). The present study examines the role of caregiver's locus of control (LOC) in education intervention for IYCF. The study aims at examining whether infant feeding and psychosocial stimulation activities motivate caregivers differently based on their LOC? Though this construct has undergone considerable elaboration and several context-specific instruments have been developed, health researchers in particular have used LOC as a concept for explaining behaviour, but its role in nutrition education leading to behaviour change has not been examined.

LOC is a concept (Rotter, 1954) originally derived from social learning theory. One of the assumptions of the social learning theory upon which LOC is based is that the behaviour of individuals in a specific situation is determined by the reinforcements they receive (ibid.). Since LOC represents how a person's decision-making ability is influenced; essentially, those who make choices on their own accord are considered to have internal loci, while those who make decisions based more on what others desire are said to have external loci. A more internal LOC is generally seen as desirable. A caregiver's perception of control may be vital in behavioural change where she can translate the knowledge she receives through education intervention into practice thereby leading to behaviour change. Examining this dimension could further help in understanding the dynamics that underpins behaviour change. It has been suggested that LOC is related to motivation, effort, performance and satisfaction (Spector, 1982).

Based on the theoretical conceptualization, individuals with an internal LOC orientation use information to more effectively control their environment. Whereas, individuals with an external LOC orientation are less likely to actively search for relevant information because they perceive that they lack control over their environment (Darley and Johnson, 1993).

The present study hypothesized that mothers with an internal LOC will have children with better growth and development compared to mothers with external LOC at the end of intervention.

METHODS AND MATERIALS

Data for the present study were collected from a three-arm cluster randomized controlled trial (Vazir et al., 2013). The mothers in this trail were recruited when their infants were three months old. Six hundred mother–infant dyads participated in the study. Sixty villages were covered so as to enrol 600 mothers and their infants. There were two intervention groups and one control group. Each group comprised 20 villages. Intervention was randomly allocated to the three arms. The intervention lasted for a period of one year.

Description of study groups and the intervention given:

1. Group 1 (standard of care): Caregivers and children in this group received the services provided by the Integrated Child Development Services (ICDS), which is a government programme. All participants in the study had access to these services. This group however received ICDS alone and served as the control group.

2. Group 2 (breastfeeding and complementary feeding): Caregivers in this group received sustained nutrition education intervention on breastfeeding and complementary feeding for a period of one year by a trained village worker.
3. Group 3 (responsive feeding and care for development): Caregivers and children in this group received education intervention on responsive feeding (UNICEF, 1997; Engle et al., 2000; PAHO/WHO, 2003) and child development stimulation combined with nutrition education on breastfeeding and complementary feeding intervention.

The study was approved by the Institutional Ethics Committee of the National Institute of Nutrition (ICMR), Hyderabad, India, and the Institutional Review Board of the University of North Carolina, USA.

INSTRUMENTS AND PROCEDURES

Maternal LOC was assessed at the end of the intervention using Rotter's (1966) LOC scale. The LOC scale has 29 pairs of items. A low score (<12) indicates an internal LOC. Test data on the Rotter's LOC scale obtained in a series of samples indicate reasonably high internal consistency estimates in the range of 0.65–0.79 (Rotter, 1972). Test–retest reliability estimates are satisfactory and are largely in the range of 0.60–0.83 (ibid.). Cronbach's alpha for the scale in the present study was 0.65. For the present study, the scale was translated to the local language. Though originally this is a self-report scale, the interview method was followed for the present study as many mothers were not literate. Each pair of statements were read out to the mothers, and they responded by choosing one of the two statements. The same procedure was followed for all the 29 pairs of statements. The scale was pretested before the data collection and this method was found to be suitable.

Infants and toddlers were weighed every month using standard Seca electronic weighing scales precise to 10 g and calibrated weekly. An infantometer with precision of 0.1 cm was used to measure supine length of infants every month. All measurement techniques including maternal height and weight at baseline followed standard approved procedures (Lohman et al., 1988). The scores were converted to z scores for analysis (Mei and Grummer-Strawn, 2007).

Child development was assessed using the Bayley's Scales of Infant Development or BSID (Bayley, 1993). The scales have been extensively used worldwide to assess the development of infants. The BSID are used to describe the current developmental functioning of infants and to assist in diagnosis and treatment planning for infants with developmental delays or disabilities.

The BSID II scales yield the Mental Developmental Index (BSID-II-MDI) and the Psychomotor Developmental Index (BSID-II-PDI), the mean BSID-II-MDI and BSID-II-PDI scores in healthy infants and children are 100 ± 15.

Since earlier studies have shown LOC to be associated with education and socio-economic status (Sennett and Cobb, 1973; Rubin, 1976; Bosma et al., 1998), these variables were also assessed. Socio-economic status of the family was assessed using a checklist of various household articles that the family owned. The checklist had 18 articles, namely (1) a mattress, (2) a pressure cooker, (3) a chair, (4) a cot or bed, (5) a table, (6) a clock or watch, (7) an electric fan, (8) a bicycle, (9) a radio or transistor, (10) a sewing machine, (11) a telephone, (12) a refrigerator, (13) a black and white television, (14) a colour television, (15) a moped, scooter, or motorcycle, (16) a water pump, (17) a bullock cart and, (18) a tractor. Each of these articles was given a score of one. The total score of these articles was converted to percentage (NFHS-3, 2005–06).

Maternal education level was categorized into illiterate, mothers with primary level of education and mothers with secondary and higher education.

Community: Caste system is prevalent in the community studied. The three caste groups are (1) the scheduled caste (SC), (2) other backward castes (OBCs) and (3) other castes (OCs). Besides the caste groups, the scheduled tribe (ST) is also present. The ST, SC and OBCs are more socially and economically disadvantaged compared to OCs.

Statistical Analyses: Descriptive statistics and analysis of variance were done using SPSS version 15.0.

Results and Discussion: Differences between groups in terms of the outcome variables of child growth and development were assessed. Comparisons of means of continuous variables were done using ANOVA and *t*-tests, chi-square tests were used for distribution of categorical variables. The anthropometry data converted to z-scores using the WHO standards.

Table 13.1 Per cent Distribution of Mothers according to Internal/External Locus of Control in the Three Study Groups

Study Groups	*Maternal LOC Scores*		*N*
	Internal <12	*External >= 12*	
1	74.1[a,b]	25.9	170
2	66.5[a]	33.5	167
3	79.2[b]	20.8	159
Pooled	73.2	26.8	496
Chi-square = 6.9			
P = <0.05			

Note: The letters a, b, c in the table relects post hoc differences between groups. Different superscript letters means the groups are significantly diffrent. Same superscript letters means the groups are not significantly different.

Table 13.1 gives the distribution of the LOC scores in the three study groups. The per cent mothers with internal LOC were higher in three study groups compared to mothers with external LOC. Post hoc test shows significant group differences, with the complimentarys feeding intervention group (group 2) having significantly lower number of *internals* compared to the control group (group 1) and the complimentary responsive feeding and care for development intervention group (group 3). Individuals with a strong *internal* LOC believe that the responsibility for whether they get reinforced or not is ultimately with them, and they believe that success or failure is due to their own efforts (Rotter, 1966). Since LOC (Rotter, 1975) is a generalized expectancy and predicts people's behaviour across situations, it can be assumed that most of the mothers in the study population would behave as *internals* in most situations. However, there may be some specific situations where people, who are generally *external,* would behave like *internals* as their learning history has shown them that they have control over the reinforcement they receive in certain situations, although overall they perceive little control over what happens to them. It is therefore important to look at these characteristics as the interaction of the person and the environment (Rotter, 1975).

The schedule caste (SC) and schedule tribe (ST) are the socially and economically disadvantaged group. Other backward caste (OBC) is in the intermediate position, whereas people from other caste (OC) are the top rung in the community hierarchy. Results (Table 13.2) show that SC/ST and OBC are significantly

Table 13.2 Means and Standard Deviations of Maternal Locus of Control Scores according to Community

Caste	*Mean*	*SD*	*N*
SC + ST	9.0[a]	2.82	127
OBC	9.7[a]	2.84	324
OC	8.8[b]	2.68	43
F value for community: 3.85, $p <.05$			

Note: Means with differing superscripts are significantly different from each other.

($p <.05$) different from OC community. The OC community had the lowest score implying a more *internal* LOC. The most disadvantaged communities have higher scores. However, all the communities come under the internal LOC category. The 'Other Caste' shows a more stronger orientation to being internally controlled, this could be owing to their standing in the community and their socio-economic status, at the same time the more disadvantaged communities do not show helplessness or lack of control over life situation as is typical with people with an external LOC. The mothers in the present study are more internally controlled.

LOC varied significantly ($p <.05$) according to mother's level of education (Table 13.3). The LOC scores of mothers with secondary and above educational level were the lowest among all other educational levels in the three study groups, indicating an internal orientation. These findings are similar to earlier findings where higher education was associated with internal LOC (Stipek and Weisz, 1981; Nunn et al., 1986). Earlier studies have also showed that students with *internal* LOC have significantly higher school achievement and were less likely to drop out of a course (Dille and Mezack, 1991; Pugliese, 1994; Njus and Brockway, 1999).

Family assets were categorized into three levels (< 33.3 per cent, 33.3–44.4 per cent and > 44.4 per cent) on the basis of per cent assets that the family possessed (Table 13.4). Results indicated that maternal LOC according to assets were not significantly different. LOC was not determined by socio-economic level (measured by number of family possessions) in the present population. The households were more or less homogenous. Other indicators of socio-economic status such as ownership of house and land holdings were not included in the present study.

Table 13.3 Mean and Standard Deviations of Maternal LOC according to Educational Level in the Three Study Groups Using ANOVA

Maternal Education	Group 1			Group 2			Group 3			Total		
	Mean	*SD*	*N*	*Mean*	*SD*	*N*	*Mean*	*SD*	*N*	*Mean*	*SD*	*N*
Illiterate	10.3^{a}	3.06	65	10.2^{a}	2.40	66	10.0^{a}	2.76	63	10.2^{a}	2.74	194
Primary	9.2^{b}	2.64	59	10.3^{b}	2.71	58	8.9^{b}	2.90	45	9.5^{b}	2.79	162
Secondary and above	8.0^{c}	2.44	46	8.9^{c}	3.35	43	8.2^{c}	2.24	49	8.3^{c}	2.70	138
Total			170			167			157			494

F value for education: 17.7; $p = <.01$.

Note: Group mean with differing superscripts is significantly different from each other.

Table 13.4 Means and Standard Deviations of Maternal LOC according to Per cent Family Assets in the Three Study Groups Using ANOVA

Family Assets (%)	*Group 1*			*Group 2*			*Group 3*			*Total*
	Mean	*SD*	*N*	*Mean*	*SD*	*N*	*Mean*	*SD*	*N*	*N*
< 33.3	9.6	2.42	51	10.0	2.49	48	9.9	2.92	53	9.8	2.62	152
33.3–44.4	9.4	2.94	47	9.4	2.65	49	8.8	2.85	43	9.2	2.80	139
> 44.4	9.0	3.16	72	10.2	3.13	70	8.6	2.39	61	9.3	3.00	203
Total			170			167			157			494

F value for assets: 2.48; p =. 09 (NS)

Table 13.5 Means and Standard Deviations of Children's Height for Age, Weight for Height and Weight for Age Z Scores according to LOC in the Three Study Groups Using ANOVA

GROUP/Maternal LOC Categories	*Stunting (Height for Age) Z Scores*		*Wasting (Weight for Height) Z Scores*		*Under-Nutrition (Weight for Age) Z Scores*		*N*
	Mean	*SD*	*Mean*	*SD*	*Mean*	*SD*	
Group 1							
Internal LOC	−1.6356	0.95769	−0.7813	1.08441	−1.3335	1.04743	122
External LOC	−1.7140	1.12580	−0.6837	1.05015	−1.3153	1.11380	43
Group 2							
Internal LOC	−1.5246	0.86616	−0.7472	1.00628	−1.2585	0.91599	108
External LOC	−1.3493	0.91322	−0.4306	0.84320	−0.9369	0.86071	54
Group 3							
Internal LOC	−1.5648	0.92820	−0.8732	0.98196	−1.3663	0.94175	120
External LOC	−1.6190	0.90656	−1.0232	0.98010	−1.5019	0.88568	31
F value	0.98	1.947	1.94				
P value	0.42	0.085	0.08				

'Wasting' (weight for height) and under-nutrition (weight for age) parameters were not significantly different but showed a trend ($p = .08$) while stunting was comparable between groups (Table 13.5). Children whose mothers had *external* LOC (Group 2 complimentary feeding intervention group) had better nutritional status compared to the children whose mother's had *internal* LOC category. There was lesser wasting and under-nutrition in Group 2 (complimentary feeding intervention). This group also had the highest percentage of mothers in the external LOC category. Though both the intervention groups received education intervention on complimentary feeding, Group 2 had children with lesser growth faltering. The fact that individuals with an external LOC orientation are less likely to actively search for relevant information because they perceive that they lack control over their environment (Darley and Johnson, 1993) could be facilitating them towards behaviour change when information is delivered to them in their homes during the home visits, and they can access this information in their own environment although the evidence for this is only marginal in terms of child growth in the present study as observed among the externals of Group 2.

Table 13.6 Means and Standard Deviations of Children's Mental and Motor Index Scores according to Maternal Internal/External LOC in the Three Study Groups ANOVA

Group/Maternal LOC	*Bayley Mental Index Scores*		*Bayley Scale Motor Index Scores*		*N*
	Mean	*SD*	*Mean*	*SD*	
Group 1					
Internal LOC	105.1[ac]	9.02	115.5	14.73	123
External LOC	103.0[c]	9.02	111.9	15.1	43
Group 2					
Internal LOC	107.4[b]	7.95	116.1	14.76	111
External LOC	103.1[c]	9.29	114.8	14.49	56
Group 3					
Internal LOC	107.8[b]	8.50	116.6	14.64	125
External LOC	106.6[ab]	6.84	116.7	13.7	33
F value	4.34		0.74		
P value	0.01		0.58		

Note: Mean with differing superscripts are significant post hoc differences between groups and maternal LOC.

Table 13.6 gives the mean Mental and Motor Index scores classified according to the maternal LOC categories. The intervention on responsive feeding and care for development intervention was given only to Group 3. The improvement in the mental index therefore was expected only in this group. But when group comparisons were made based on *internal* and *external* LOC categories, results show that the *internals* of both Group 2 and Group 3 had the same mean score that was higher than Group 1—the control group. A similar trend was not seen in the *externals*. In this category Group 1 and Group 2 *external* category had lower mean scores (103 DQ points) where as the *externals* who received the intervention had a mean DQ of 106. These results show that mother's *internal* LOC is beneficial for the mental development for the child (*internal* category have better mean DQ scores in all the groups). These results also show that with intervention, the externals catch up with the internals. Here again, the same trend was observed as in growth, in that externals benefit relatively more when compared to internals from an education intervention. These differences are small, yet they can be insightful in explaining why most of the education intervention trials show only modest improvement. One reason could possibly be that the populations are more skewed towards being *internal;* these individuals already have a mind set that they control their environment and so seek out information even before any interventions are implemented or at their own will. Externals on the other hand (1/4 of the total sample in the present study) get an opportunity to receive information in their own environment; only through these types of interventions they also seem to comply with the education given to them, and therefore show more improvement. Since they form a smaller part of the sample the improvements seen are also relatively low.

The results also show that with intervention mothers learn and provide stimulation to their children such that their development is comparable to children whose mothers have internal LOC this confirms the benefit of the intervention.

Rotter has written extensively on problems with people's interpretations of the LOC concept that it is not a typology. It is not an either/or proposition. Since it is a generalized expectancy, it will predict people's behaviour across situations. However, in certain situations people may behave differently based on their previous learning, for example, people, who are generally external, behave like internals. In an education intervention when 'do able' advise, problem solving and motivation are used; mothers with external LOC are likely to practice it, empowering them to take on responsibility. In these situations, they behave like *internals,* but their overall general expectancy is still that of an *external*. Further research will be necessary to establish LOC as a predictor of success of education interventions.

Since the data for this study were taken from a larger study, the groups had lesser number of externals when compared to internals; while this is a limitation of the study, it also showed that most of the rural mothers have an internal LOC.

REFERENCES

Aruna, M., S. Vazir and P. Vidyasagar, 2001, 'Child Rearing and Positive Deviance in the Development of Preschool Children: A Micro Analysis', *Indian Paediatrics*, 38: 332–39.

Bayley, N., 1993, *Bayley Scales of Infant Development*, 2nd ed. (BSID-II). San Antonio, TX: The Psychological Corporation.

Bhandari, Nita, Sarmila Mazumder, Rajiv Bahl, Jose Martines, Robert E. Black, Maharaj K. Bhan, 2004, 'An Educational Intervention to Promote Appropriate Complementary Feeding Practices and Physical Growth in Infants and Young Children in Rural Haryana, India', *The Journal of Nutrition*, 134(9): 2342–48.

Bosma, H., H.D. Van de Mheen and J.P. Mackenbach, 1998, 'Childhood Socioeconomic Conditions and Adult Health: The Contribution of Psychological Attributes'. Presented at the International Congress of Behavioural Medicine, Copenhagen, Denmark, 21 August.

Darley, W. and D. Johnson, 1993, 'Effects of Female Adolescent Locus of Control on Shopping Behaviour, Fashion Orientation and Information Search', *International Review of Retail, Distribution, and Consumer Research*, 3: 149–65.

Dille, B. and M. Mezack, 1991, 'Identifying Predictors of High Risk Among Community College Telecourse Students', *The American Journal of Distance Education*, 2(1): 25–37.

Engle, P.L., M. Bentley and G. Pelto, 2000, 'The Role of Care in Nutrition Programmes: Current Research and a Research Agenda', *Proceedings of the Nutrition Society*, 59: 25–35.

Guldan, Georgia S., Heng-Chun Fan, Xiao Ma, Zong-Zan Ni, Xia Xiang and Ming-Zhen Tang, 2000, 'Culturally Appropriate Nutrition Education Improves Infant Feeding and Growth in Rural Sichuan, China', *Journal of Nutrition*, 130: 1204–11.

Lohman, T.G., A.F. Roche and R. Martorell, 1988, *Anthropometric Standardization Reference Manual*. Champaign, IL: Human Kinetics Books.

Mei, Z. and L.M. Grummer-Strawn, 2007, 'Standard Deviation of Anthropometric Z-Scores as a Data Quality Assessment Tool Using 2006 WHO Growth Standards', *Bulletin of the World Health Organization*, 85(6): 421–500.

Njus, D.M. and J.H. Brockway, 1999, 'Perceptions of Competence 8c Locus of Control for Positive and Negative Outcomes', *Personality and Individual Differences*, 26: 531–48.

Nunn, G.D., J.D. Montgomery and S.J. Nunn, 1986, 'Criterion-Related Validity of the Nowicki-Strickland Locus of Control Scale with Academic Achievement', *Psychology: A Quarterly Journal of Human Behaviour*, 23: 9–11.

PAHO/World Health Organization, 2003, *Guiding Principles for Complementary Feeding of the Breastfed Child*. Geneva, Switzerland: PAHO/WHO, World Health Organization.

Pugliese, R.R., 1994, 'Telecourse Persistence and Psychological Variables', *American Journal of Distance Education*, 8(3): 2239.

Rotter, J.B., 1954, *Social Learning and Clinical Psychology*. Englewood Cliffs, NJ: Prentice Hall.

Rotter, J.B., 1966, 'Generalized Expectancies for Internal versus External Control of Reinforcement', *Psychological Monographs*, 80(1, Whole No. 609).

Rotter, J.B., 1972, 'Generalized Expectancies for Internal versus External Control of Reinforcements'. In *Applications of a Social Learning Theory of Personality*, edited by, J.B. Rotter, J.E. Chance and E.J. Phares, New York: Holt, Rinehart & Winston.

Rotter, J.B., 1975, 'Some Problems and Misconceptions Related to the Construct of Internal versus External Control of Reinforcement', *Journal of Consulting and Clinical Psychology*, 43: 56–67.Rubin, L.B., 1976, *Worlds of Pain*. New York: Basic Books.

Sennett, R. and J. Cobb, 1973, *The Hidden Injuries of Class*. New York: Vintage Books.

Spector, Paul E., 1982, 'Behavior in Organizations as a Function of Employee's Locus of Control', *Psychological Bulletin*, 91(3): 482–97.

Stipek, D. and J. Weisz, 1981, 'Perceived Personal Control and Academic Achievement', *Review of Educational Research*, 51: 101–37.

UNICEF, 1997, *The Care Initiative Assessment, Analysis, and Action to Improve Care for Nutrition*. New York: UNICEF Nutrition Section.

Vazir, Shahnaz, Patrice Engle, Nagalla Balakrishna, Paula L. Griffiths, Susan L. Johnson, Hilary Creed-Kanashiro, Sylvia Fernandez Rao, Monal R. Shroff and Margaret E. Bentley, 2013, 'Cluster-Randomized Trial on Complementary and Responsive Feeding Education to Caregivers Found Improved Dietary Intake, Growth and Development Among Rural Indian Toddlers', *Maternal and Child Nutrition*, 9: 99–117.

Wachs, T.D., H. Creed-Kanashiro, S. Cueto and E. Jacoby, 2005, 'Maternal Education and Intelligence Predict Offspring Diet and Nutritional Status', *Journal of Nutrition*, 135: 2179–86.

CHAPTER 14

Health Status of Pregnant Women among Scheduled Castes in Madurai District of Tamil Nadu

M. Thamilarasan and M. Suganya

INTRODUCTION

Maternal and child health (MCH) have remained an integral part of the Family Welfare Programme of India since the time of the First and Second Five-Year Plans (1951–56 and 1956–61) when the Government of India took steps to strengthen MCH services. As part of the Minimum Needs Programme initiated during the fifth Five-Year Plan (1974–79), maternal health, child health and nutrition services were integrated with family planning services. In 1992–93, the Child Survival and Safe Motherhood Programme continued the process of integration by bringing together several key child survival interventions with safe motherhood and family planning activities. In 1996, safe motherhood and child health services were incorporated into the Reproductive and Child Health Programme (RCH). The National Population Policy adopted by the Government of India in 2000 reiterates the government's commitment to safe motherhood programmes within the wider context of reproductive health. Several national socio-demographic goals for 2010 specified by the policy pertain to safe motherhood. For 2010, the goals are that 80 per cent of all deliveries should take place in institutions, 100 per cent of deliveries should be attended by trained personnel and the maternal mortality ratio should be reduced to a level below 100 per 100,000 live births.

In order to improve the availability of and access to quality health care, especially for those residing in rural areas, the poor, women and children, the government recently launched the National Rural Health Mission for the 2005–2012 periods. One of the important goals of the National Rural Health Mission is to provide access to improved health care at the household level through female Accredited Social Health Activists (ASHA), who act as an interface between the community and the public health system. The ASHA acts as a bridge between the auxiliary nurse midwife (ANM) and the village, and she is accountable to the *panchayat*. She helps promote referrals for universal immunization, escort services for RCH, construction of household toilets and other health care delivery programmes.

Concept and Definition of Pregnancy

Medical dictionary by FARLEX defines pregnancy as

> The period from conception to birth. After the egg is fertilized by a sperm and then implanted in the lining of the uterus, it develops into the placenta and embryo, and later into fetus. Pregnancy usually last 40 weeks, beginning from the first day of the woman's last menstrual period, and is divided into 3 trimesters, each lasting 3 times. (http://medical-dictionary.thefreedictionary.com/pregnancy)

Pregnancy is the carrying of one or more offspring, known as a foetus or embryo, in the womb of a woman. In a pregnancy, there can be multiple gestations, as in the case of twins or triplets. Childbirth usually occurs about 38 weeks after conception; in women who have a menstrual cycle length of four weeks, this is nearly 40 weeks from the last normal menstrual period. The World Health Organization (WHO) defines normal term for delivery as between 37 and 42 weeks. Human pregnancy is the most studied of all mammalian pregnancies.

One scientific term for the state of pregnancy is gravidity (adjective 'gravid'), and a pregnant female is sometimes referred to as a gravida. Neither word is used in common speech. Similarly, the term 'parity' (abbreviated as 'para') is used for the number of previous successful live births. Medically, a woman who has never been pregnant is referred to as a 'nulligravida', a woman who is (or has been only) pregnant for the first time as a 'primigravida', and a woman in subsequent pregnancies as a multigravida or 'multiparous'.

WHO's Definition of Health

The widely accepted definition of health is given by the WHO (2001): Health is a state of complete physical, mental and social well-being, and not merely an absence of disease or infirmity.

The WHO definition has been criticized, as 'health' cannot be defined as a 'state', but it is a dynamic concept subjected to change with regard to age, sex, environment, etc. Hence, WHO definition is considered by many as an idealistic goal than a realistic proposition. Despite its above limitations, it sets out the standard, the standard for 'positive health', which represents overall goal towards which each nation should strive for.

DIMENSION OF HEALTH

Physical Dimension

This dimension is very easily understandable. It denotes perfect functioning of the body. The general signs of physical health are: A well built body, with firm flesh, clean skin, lustrous hair, with bright eyes; good appetite, good sleep, regular bowel habits, bladder movement normal; all the organs of the body normal and functioning normally; all senses are intact; the pulse rate, blood pressure are within normal range, with reference to age, and sex; the height and weight are normal.

These parameters can be easily assessed by various techniques.

Mental Dimension

A person mentally healthy will have the characteristics such as adjustable in nature; interact with others, free from internal conflicts, self-consciousness, self-control and intelligent in tackling problems, which he faces. The stated characteristics cannot be easily assessed by any physical methods. Unfortunately, our knowledge about mental health is far from complete.

Social Dimension

Social health is a condition in which an individual can lead a healthy living as a member of the society. It is the status of community, which ensures healthy living of the members of community, in a social set-up. The social harmony and the economical inputs in social well-being all attribute to social well-being. All social needs such as protected water, clean environment, material benefits and social harmony attribute to social dimension. In other words, it is a social condition in which a willing individual is able to maintain a physical and mental well-being without any difficulty.

Spiritual Dimension

Though it is not mentioned by WHO, many aspire to induct this 'spiritual concept', which enables humans to realize their purpose of living; although it is a newer concept, in modern days, its realization is very much felt, as humans tend to derail from moral path, as science advances.

It is not a religious concept, rather it is a concept by which it exposes humans to integrity and ethics and helps them to lead a purposeful life, which elevates them to the higher planes of thought.

Other Dimensions

There are other dimensions, such as economical, educational and philosophical, and all of them contribute only to the physical, mental and social well-being.

Women's health is harmed by lack of access to and the poor quality of reproductive services. About 24.6 million couples, representing roughly eighteen per cent of all married women, want no more children but are not using contraception. The causes of this unmet need remain poorly understood, but a qualitative study in Tamil Nadu suggests that women's lack of decision making power in the family, opportunity costs involved in seeking contraception, fear of child death and poor quality of contraceptive service all play an important role.

Some estimates suggest that some five million abortions are performed annually in India, with the large majority being illegal. As a result, abortion-related mortality is high. Although abortion has been legal since 1972 in India, studies suggest that although official policy seeks to make pregnancy-termination services widely available, in practice guidelines on abortion limit access to services, particularly in rural areas.

The tasks performed by women are usually those that require them to be in one position for long periods of time, which adversely affect their reproductive health. A study in a rice-growing belt of coastal Maharashtra found that 40 per cent of all infant deaths occurred in the months of July through October. The study also found that a majority of births were either premature or stillbirths. The study attributed this to the squatting position that had to be assumed during July and August, the rice-transplanting months.

REVIEW OF LITERATURE

Velkoff and Adlakha (1998) published that over 100,000 Indian women die each year from pregnancy-related causes. Maternal mortality and morbidity are two health concerns that are related to high levels of fertility. India has a high maternal mortality ratio, nearly 453 deaths per 100,000 births in 1993. This ratio is 57 times the ratio in the United States. The World Health Organization (WHO) and United Nations Children's Fund (UNICEF) estimates that India's maternal mortality is lower than ratios for Bangladesh and Nepal but higher than those for Pakistan and Sri Lanka in 1996. The level of maternal mortality varies greatly by state, with Kerala having the lowest ratio (87) and two states (Madhya Pradesh and Orissa) having ratio over 700. This differential maternal mortality is most likely related to differences in the social economic status of women. The high levels of maternal mortality are especially distressing because the majority of these deaths could be prevented if women had adequate health services.

Kwalombota (2002) says that AIDS is a formidable problem in sub-Saharan African countries, including Angola. In his findings, two-thirds of HIV-positive pregnant women had significant emotional distress; it corroborates with the findings from studies in other populations showing that the majority of HIV-positive pregnant women suffer from poor mental health.

UNDP (1998) stated that in the past, traditional faith healers and traditional birth attendants provided health care in Nepal. It was during the end of the nineteenth century that the concept of modern medicine was introduced in Nepal. Starting from the mid-1950s, planned national level efforts towards the development of modern health services were initiated. Since then, progress has been made in the development of modern health services, and in recent years, modern health care has penetrated various parts of Nepal. However, the services are still limited in number; especially in remote rural areas, at present, both modern and traditional forms of medicine coexist simultaneously in the country.

UNICEF (2006) stated that in Nepal, the prevailing attitude towards pregnancy is that it is not considered the condition that requires special treatment. Therefore, antenatal care (ANC) and medical care are not considered essential components of pregnancy. In addition, for cultural reasons, women are reluctant to seek ANC especially from male health worker. Consequently, in some cases, even when adequate services are available women are reluctant to use them.

Naik (2011) says that some 1,400 women die every day from problems related to pregnancy and childbirth. The dangers of childbearing can be greatly reduced if a woman is healthy and well-nourished before becoming pregnant and if she has regular health check-up during pregnancy.

To have safe motherhood:

1. It is important for all families to be able to recognize the warning signs of problems during pregnancy and childbirth and to have plans and resources for getting immediate skilled help if problems arise. A pregnant woman needs to be checked at a clinic or health facility at least four times during every pregnancy. Risk factors before pregnancy have to be checked such as an interval of less than two years since an earlier birth. Consider a girl under 18 years or a woman above 35 years of age. The woman already has four or more children. The woman has had a previous premature birth or baby weighing less than 2 kg at birth. The woman has had a previous miscarriage or stillbirth. The woman weighs less than 38 kg. Warning signs during pregnancy are failure to gain weight (at least 6 kg should be gained during pregnancy), anaemia, paleness inside the eyelids, very tired or easily out of breath, unusual swelling of legs, arms or face. The foetus moves very little or does not move at all. The following are the signs that need help immediately: spotting or bleeding from the vagina during pregnancy or profuse or persistent bleeding after delivery, severe headache or stomach ache, severe/persistent vomiting, high fever, the water breaks before due time for delivery, convulsions, severe pain, prolonged labour.

2. A skilled birth attendant, such as a doctor, nurse/trained midwife should check the woman at least four times during every pregnancy and assist at every birth. If any of the warning signs

does occur, a health worker/skilled birth attendant should be consulted immediately. A skilled birth attendant (such as a doctor, nurse/trained midwife) will help to ensure a safer pregnancy and healthy baby by checking the progress of pregnancy, checking for high blood pressure, checking for anaemia, checking for any infections, giving two injections against tetanus, encourage all pregnant women to use only iodized salt, advise on breast feeding and care if new born.

3. All pregnant women need particularly nutritious meals and more rest than usual throughout pregnancy.
4. A pregnant woman needs the best foods available to family: milk, fruits, vegetables, meat, fish, eggs, grains, peas and beans. Women will feel stronger and healthier during pregnancy if they eat foods that are rich in iron, vitamin A and folic acid. Health workers can provide them with iron tablets to prevent or treat anaemia. Salt should be iodized.
5. Smoking, alcohol, drugs, poisons and pollutants are especially harmful to pregnant women and young children. To ensure physical growth and mental development of the child, pregnant women and young children need to be protected from tobacco smoke or cooking fire, from pesticides and other poisons.
6. Physical abuse of women and children is a serious public health problem in many communities. Abuse during pregnancy is dangerous to both the woman and the foetus. Physically abused pregnant women may be unable to have any more children. Family members should protect her from her abuser.
7. Girls who are educated, healthy and have a good diet during their childhood and teenage (teenagers) will have fewer problems in pregnancy and childbirth.

Girls who have at least seven years of schooling are less likely to become pregnant during adolescence and are more likely to marry later than those with little or no education.

Mercer et al. (2006) stated that Bangladesh is fairly typical of low-income countries, with neonatal mortality accounting for about two-thirds of deaths among infants and about half of deaths among children younger than five years. Data from the management information system, a large non-governmental organization (NGO) programme, in rural Bangladesh indicate that the NMR in the NGO served areas declined from 39 deaths per 1,000 live births in 1996 to 20 per 1,000 live births in 2002 through programme called Bangladesh Population and Health Consortium. It studied 12 sub-districts distributed across 12 different districts about 580,000 people in 1,050,000 households. The programme includes the service and checks related to neonatal deaths, use of reproductive health outreach services (antenatal and postnatal care, attendance at delivery, family planning and tetanus toxoid immunization).

UNFPA (2002) says that pregnancy and motherhood are among the most important gender roles fulfilled by women throughout the world. It is unfortunate, however, that pregnancy and childbirth may be the only events that bring women into sustained contact with the health care system in any number of developing countries. MCH programmes (i.e. antenatal, delivery and postpartum services) therefore provide a unique opportunity to reach women at risk or otherwise vulnerable to HIV infection with critical information, technological and services.

Voluntary HIV counselling and testing in antenatal clinics is particularly important for pregnant women because a diagnosis of HIV infection is the only way to ensure access to the growing number of interventions designed to prevent the transmission of the virus to their newly born children, including access to drug therapies such as zidovudine and nevirapine. Another important reason to integrate voluntary counselling and testing programmes into antenatal clinics is the opportunity it provides for reaching husbands and male partners of pregnant women. Pregnancy can increase men's and, subsequently, women's vulnerability to STIs and HIV. Because cultural and other factors and social stigmas limit sexual activity between couples during pregnancy and the postpartum period, men are likely to seek outside partners during that time (Lawoyin and Larsen, 2002).

Kulkarni et al. (1996) conducted a five year study of maternal mortality due to jaundice, in Bellary, Karnataka, during the period 1991–95. It is retrospective hospital-based study and aims to analyse maternal deaths due to jaundice. Retrospective analysis of all maternal deaths occurring during the study period due to jaundice was carried out. Twenty-three maternal deaths were due to jaundice from the study group.

The researcher found in the study that there were a total of 12,723 deliveries, of which 223 ended in maternal deaths, giving a maternal mortality ratio of 1,752 per 100,000 live births. Jaundice accounted for 23 maternal deaths, or 10.4 per cent of all maternal deaths and 30 per cent of all maternal deaths from indirect cause (there were 77 maternal deaths from indirect causes). There were 82 jaundice patients in all. Thus, 28 per cent of the proportion of deaths due to jaundice was 23 of 82. A total of 15 of the 23 deaths occurred in women who were more than 28 weeks pregnant (9 deaths) or in the puerperium (6 deaths), 7 deaths were in women who were in the 21–27 week, of gestation and only one death occurred in a woman who was less than 20 weeks pregnant. Of the 23, 15 were admitted with jaundice, where as 8 were admitted without jaundice. A total of 14 died after delivery of which 7 had stillbirths. Of the 14, 7 had premature labour and 7 delivered near term. In 2, the outcome was abortion while 7 died before delivery. The majority of the patients died within one to three days after admission. A total of 14 of 23 died due to hepatic coma, 3 died due to postpartum haemorrhage and hepato-renal failure, 2 died due to sepsis and 1 due to imbolism.

Sravani (2011) says that over-the-counter (OTC) drug should be avoided in pregnancy. OTC drugs are medicines that may be sold directly to a consumer without a prescription from a health care professional. OTC medicines are used many times to relieve pain and treat the symptoms of common cold and allergies. But like prescription drugs, OTC medicines can also cause unwanted and sometimes dangerous side effects one needs to be aware of. Some of the best-known medicines from the local drug store can be harmful to pregnant women, yet many mothers-to-be regularly take them.

The problem caused by medicines taken by the mother is that they can cross the placenta and enter the baby's bloodstream. This is because the medicine particles are small enough to cross the placental barrier along with the nutrients needed for the baby's development. The effect any medicine has on the developing baby depends on the medicine itself and the trimester of pregnancy the medicine is taken in.

Sujatha (2003) explained about medical lore. The knowledge and practice of the common people in villages, pertaining to health, disease and medicine, is what we call medical lore. 'Knowledge', in this definition, is particularly important because it normally does not figure in most references to folklore on health. References to the health traditions of the village folk employ terms such as 'beliefs', 'superstitions', 'magic' and 'habits', not even ideas. Anthropologists and scholars on health policy, who are the people to study folk medical systems, have perceived medical lore only as a bundle of magical beliefs, superstitions and some remedies.

Florez and Hogan (1990) stated that in Asia partly owing to the low utilization of maternal health services, particular focus was given in the article to women's status and household structures while controlling for the accessibility factor. It has been argued that changes in women's status have been the key to differentiate the behaviour of those seeking for themselves and their children modern health care from those following traditional practices.

RESEARCH METHODOLOGY

Statement of the Problem

The present study titled 'Health status of pregnant women among schedule caste in Madurai district of Tamil Nadu' is an attempt to analyse the health condition of pregnant women. The study also involves the food pattern of the pregnant women, which has an influence on their health status during pregnancy. It studies the changes that are occurring during pregnancy and the level of awareness they possess about their own health condition during pregnancy.

ANC refers to pregnancy-related health care, which is usually provided by a doctor, an ANM or another health professional. Ideally, ANC should monitor a pregnancy for signs of complications, detect and treat pre-existing and concurrent problems of pregnancy, and provide advice and counselling on preventive care, diet during pregnancy, delivery care, postnatal care and related issues. In India, the RCH aims at providing at least three antenatal check-ups, which should include a weight and blood pressure check, abdominal examination, immunization against tetanus, iron and folic acid prophylaxis, as well as anaemia management.

NFHS-3 collected information from women on specific problems they may have had during their pregnancies and whether they saw anyone for ANC for their pregnancy. Women who received ANC were asked about the care provider, the timing of the first ANC visit, the total number of visits, the procedures conducted as part of their ANC and the advice given to them. In addition, the survey asked women whether they received tetanus toxoid injections and iron and folic acid tablets or syrup during the pregnancy. Results from each of these questions are discussed in this chapter. The fathers of children for whom the mother did not receive ANC were asked why the mother did not receive it.

For the most recent birth in the five years preceding the survey, the mother was asked if at any time during the pregnancy she experienced any of the following pregnancy-related problems: difficulty with vision during daylight, night blindness, convulsions (not from fever), swelling of the legs, body or face, excessive fatigue or vaginal bleeding. Night blindness or difficulty in seeing at dusk is the result of chronic vitamin A deficiency and is often seen in pregnant women in areas where vitamin A deficiency is endemic. Convulsions accompanied by signs of hypertension can be symptomatic of eclampsia, a potentially fatal condition. The potential health risk posed by vaginal bleeding during pregnancy varies by when in the pregnancy the bleeding takes place. Although documenting the prevalence of the symptoms of pregnancy complications is vital for planning services to reduce maternal morbidity and mortality, the information presented here is based on women's self-reports and should be interpreted with care.

Objectives of the Study

1. To study the health status of pregnant women
2. To bring out the influence of food pattern on the health status of pregnant women
3. To find out the medical treatment of the pregnant women during pregnancy
4. To assess the awareness of pregnant women on their own health condition
5. To know the work participation of pregnant women during pregnancy

Research Design

The research design of the present study is descriptive type in which an attempt is made to discover or identify significant correlates of a social phenomenon under study, since the focus is on the health status of pregnant women among schedule caste.

Universe of the Study

Since the present study is concentrating on the health condition of pregnant women with the influence of health services, health behaviour, health practice, the researcher decided to conduct the study in Madurai city. This city is popularly known as the temple city. The city consists of different categories of people such as backward class, most backward class, scheduled caste (SC) and scheduled tribe (ST). The city has all types of health care centres ranging from primary health care centre to multi-specialty hospitals. Considering the limitation of the time and manpower, the researcher selected only one Integrated Counselling and Testing Centre (ICTC), which offers health care services to children and pregnant women. The centre (ICTC) covers three major areas of the Madurai city.

Profile of the Study Area

The total population of Tamil Nadu, as per the 2001 Census, is 62,405,679. Of this, 11,857,504 (19 per cent) are SCs. The SC population constitutes 7.1 per cent of the country's SC population. Seventy-six SCs have been notified in Tamil Nadu by the Scheduled Castes and Scheduled Tribes Order (Amendment) Act, 1976. Of these, 15 SCs, namely Ayyanavar, Bharatar, Kakkalan, Kavara, Kootan, Mannan, Padannan, Panan, Paravan, Pathiyan, Thandan, Vannan, Vetan and Vettuvan have been notified with area restriction in Kanniyakumari district and Shencottah taluk of Tirunelveli district. Kanakkan have been notified in Nilgiri district only. Out of 76 SCs, two SCs, that is Kakkalan and Padannan, have not reported population in 2001 Census.

The growth rate of SC population in the decade 1991–2001 at 10.7 per cent is lower in comparison to the overall growth rate of 11.7 per cent of the state. Among major SCs, Paraiyan have recorded the highest growth rate of 38.6 per cent, followed by Arunthathiyar (33.2 per cent) and Pallan (18.5 per cent) during 1991–2001.

Population Size and Distribution

Out of 76 SCs, 5 SCs, Adi Dravida, Pallan, Paraiyan, Chakkiliyan and Arunthathiyar, together constitute 93.5 per cent of the SC population of the state. Adi Dravida are numerically the largest SCs with a population of 5,402,755, constituting 45.6 per cent of the state's SC population. They are followed by Pallan 2,272,265 (19.2 per cent),

Paraiyan 1,860,519 (15.7 per cent), Chakkiliyan 777,139 (6.6 per cent) and Arunthathiyar 771,659 (6.5 per cent). Thirty-five SCs have reported population below one thousand. Among the districts, Thiruvarur has the highest proportion of SC population to its total population (32.4 per cent) while Kanyakumari has the lowest (4 per cent).

As per 2001 Census, 70.1 per cent of the SCs are living in the rural areas and 29.9 per cent in the urban areas of the state. Among the major SCs, Pallan have the highest (76 per cent) rural population, followed by Paraiyan (73.1 per cent), Adi Dravida (69.4 per cent), Chakkiliyan (67.9 per cent) and Arunthathiyar (64.4 per cent) (Source: Office of the Registrar General, India).

Sex Ratio

The overall sex ratio of the SC population in Tamil Nadu is 999 females per 1,000 males, which is higher than the national average of 936 for the SC population in 2001. The sex ratio of SC population has registered improvement over 978 reported in 1991 Census. Among the districts, the highest sex ratio (1059) is recorded in Tirunelveli district and the lowest in Salem district (947). At the individual caste level, all the major SCs, except Pallan and Paraiyan, have registered overall lower sex ratio compared with the state average.

As may be seen from the statement above, the child sex ratio (0–6) among the SC population of Tamil Nadu is also higher than the national SC population in the corresponding age group. In case of child sex ratio, the position of Paraiyan and Adi Dravida is even better than the rest of state SC population. However, Arunthathiyar, which is comparatively an urbanized SC community, has recorded a lower child sex ratio of 928.

Literacy and Educational Level

Literacy and level of education are two basic indicators of the level of development achieved by a group/society. Literacy results in more awareness besides contributing to the overall improvement of health, hygiene and other social conditions.

According to the 2001 Census, percentage of SC literate persons (those who can read and write with understanding) aged seven years and above is 63.2 per cent, which is lower than 73.5 per cent reported for the state as a whole. The literacy data show that the SC population of the state has made significant improvement during the decade 1991–2001.

The literacy rate, which was 46.7 per cent in 1991, increased by 16.5 percentage points in 2001.

Among the major SCs, Paraiyan are reported to have the highest literacy rate of 65.9 per cent, followed by Adi Dravida (65.3 per cent), Pallan (65 per cent), Arunthathiyar (53.7 per cent) and Chakkiliyan (50.9 per cent). The female literacy rate of 53 per cent among SC population is lower compared with 64.4 per cent among females of the state. As in literacy rate, the highest and lowest female literacy rates of 55.4 per cent and 40.8 per cent have also been recorded among Adi Dravida and Chakkiliyan.

Out of the total literates, 29 per cent are literates either without any educational level or have attained below primary level. The literates, who have attained education up to primary and middle levels, constitute 31.9 per cent and 18.4 per cent, respectively. A total of 17.4 per cent are having educational level up to matric/higher secondary, etc., levels, implying that every sixth SC literate is a matriculate. Literates with educational level of graduation and above are 2.7 per cent. Individually, Adi Dravida and Pallan (3 per cent each) have highest percentage of graduation and above educational levels.

Madurai district is one of the important districts of Tamil Nadu. The district has 13 blocks. The total land area of the district is 3,696 sq km. As per the 2001 Census, the population of Madurai district is about 26 lakhs, and it constitutes 4 per cent of the state's population. The sex ratio of the district is 978 females per 1,000 male population.

According to 2001 Census, the population is 25.8 lakhs out of which 13.0 lakh are males and 12.8 lakh are females. About 56 per cent of the population of the district lives in urban areas. The sex distribution of the population shows that 5.7 lakh are males and 5.6 lakh are females in rural areas. In urban areas, the male and female populations are 7.3 lakh and 7.1 lakh, respectively. The proportion of SCs and STs is 12.7 per cent and 6.9 per cent of the urban population and 19.7 per cent of the rural population.

As per the health department statistics, 68 maternal deaths were reported in Madurai district in 2010–11, whereas the maternal mortality figure in 2009–10 was 53. The district recorded a maternal mortality rate of 1.2 per 1,000 live births, which was higher than the state average of 0.9. The district health authorities have now swung into action to reduce pregnancy and delivery-related deaths by instructing the medical officers to take precautionary steps and create awareness among women and adolescent girls as well.

'We will set right the lacuna by analysing block-wise statistics. The first priority for us is to control anaemia as it is one of the main causes for maternal death. Pregnant women identified as high-risk cases by doctors will be given special attention', V. Shanmugasundaram, Deputy Director of Health Services, Madurai district, told *The Hindu* here on Sunday, 5 June 2011.

The maternal death figure of 68 is for the whole district including Government Rajaji Hospital (45), private nursing homes (13) and deaths during transit (7). Following the directions given by the Directorate of Public Health, the district health authorities are evolving strategies for prevention and control of maternal deaths.

R. Abdul Kareem, Assistant Director (Health), gave the break-up of how the 68 maternal deaths took place. Sixteen women died during pregnancy while one lost her life during actual delivery.

In the postnatal period, 51 women died in Madurai district after delivering a child. Maternity period lasts for 42 days after delivery. Reasons for deaths were postpartum haemorrhage, pregnancy-induced hypertension and aspiration with cardiac arrest.

One consolation for the district health authorities was that not a single maternal death occurred in the Primary Health Centres in 2010–11 even though the number of deliveries had gone up substantially in recent years.

'We identify the high risk mothers and refer them to Government Rajaji Hospital or other government hospitals while they come for check up to the PHCs. Safe delivery and good training for staff nurses are our objectives', said Dr Shanmughasundaram. The health department is intensely focusing on anaemia control as it is a prime reason for maternal death. Iron tablets and iron injections for pregnant women are being given. Maternal audit for the entire district is done periodically and medical officers' review meetings are conducted here each month.

'Anaemia has to be corrected even before marriage and it should start from adolescent girls. Pre-marital intervention for checking anaemia is the ideal way to prevent a maternal death', the Deputy Director explained. Block-wise report of Madurai district for 2010–11 has indicated that 11 maternal deaths took place in Madurai East block-Kallandhiri area. In Tirupparankundram, maternal deaths during this period were six; whereas in Alanganallur block, there were five maternal deaths.

Officials said that the Madurai Corporation area had 16 maternal deaths, whereas Chellampatti block had five deaths during the same period.

The officials' advice for pregnant women is that they should be alert when the delivery due date approaches, and it is better if they get admitted to hospital or Primary Healthcare Centre (PHC) a day or two before the due date given by doctor.

One step contemplated by the public health authorities of Madurai district is to have a tie-up and link with the '108' ambulance service by giving the particulars of delivery due dates/high-risk cases of pregnant women. 'By doing this, village health nurses and local health staff will be in touch with the 108 ambulance service so that the women can be shifted to hospital well in advance for delivery without delay. Maternal deaths during transit can also be avoided,' Dr Shanmughasundaram observed (*The Hindu*, Online edition of India's National Newspaper, Sunday, 5 June 2011).

Health Infrastructure

As on June 2008, Madurai district has 314 sub-centres and 42 primary health centres. Among them, 29 were 24 × 7 PHCs and 13 were block PHCs. Indian Public Health Standards (IPHS) facility survey was carried out in all the sub-centres and PHCs. In addition to this, one district hospital, six first referral units, three mobile medical units, five sub-divisional hospitals and 16 AYUSH hospitals were functioning in Madurai. IPHS facility survey was not carried out in these facilities. New buildings were under construction in three PHCs and two sub-divisional hospitals. Five private hospitals (more than 30 bedded) were allocated in Madurai district. IPHS upgradation was not completed. There are 1 district hospital, 5 sub-divisional hospitals, 1 community health centre (CHC), 42 PHCs, 17 public maternity homes and 4 other public sector hospitals such as Medical College hospital, SI and Railway, available in this district for delivery services. Among them, all the PHCs (42), public maternity homes (17) and other public sector hospitals such as eight ESI provide Basic Emergency Obstetric Care. District hospital (1) and sub-divisional hospitals (2) provide comprehensive emergency and obstetric care, that is having blood storage, anaesthetist and gynaecologist, with newborn care unit. Private health facilities were not accredited for Janani Suraksh Yojana (JSY).

Human Resources

As far as human resources are concerned, at the district level 104 medical officers were sanctioned and all the posts were regular in position. Separate information regarding number of gynaecologists, anaesthetists, paediatricians and other specialists were not available. On the whole, 138 staff nurses were sanctioned, among them 136 were regular in position. Forty-eight ANM posts were sanctioned as regular in position.

Rogi Kalyan Samities and Janani Suraksha Yojana

Rogi Kalyan Samities (RKS) were registered in the district hospital; all the sub-divisional hospitals (5), CHCs (1) and PHCs (42) are functioning. Initiative on public–private partnership was not undertaken in the district for the implementation of JSY scheme. Totally 20,929 institutional deliveries were reported during 2007–08. The number of women registered under JSY during 2007–08 was 10,978. Among them nearly one-fourth (23 per cent) were SC/ST and three-fourth (77 per cent) belonged to the general population. Ninety-two per cent (10,075) of the registered JSY women opted for institutional deliveries during 2007–08. Among them 23 per cent (2,259) were SC/ST women.

The SCs, also known as the Dalit, and the STs are two groupings of historically disadvantaged people who are given express recognition in the Constitution of India. During the period of British rule in the Indian sub-continent, they were known as the depressed classes.

The SCs and STs make up around 15 per cent and 7.5 per cent, respectively, of the population of India, or around 24 per cent altogether, according to the 2001 Census. The proportion of SCs and STs in the country's population has steadily risen since independence in 1947.

The Constitution (SCs) Order, 1950, lists 1,108 castes across 25 states in its First Schedule, while the Constitution (STs) Order, 1950, lists 744 tribes across 22 states in its First Schedule.

Since independence, the SCs have benefited by the 'Reservation' policy. This policy became an integral part of the Constitution through the efforts of Dr Bhimrao Ambedkar, regarded as the father of the Indian Constitution, who participated in round table conferences and fought for the rights of the depressed classes. The Constitution lays down general principles for the policy of affirmative action for the SCs and STs.

SAMPLE SELECTION

The pregnant women samples were purposefully selected from the ICTC. From this centre, 100 samples were selected. Hence, the sample size for the present study is 100.

TOOLS OF DATA COLLECTION

As soon as the topic of the research was finalized, the researcher made visits to various libraries in universities and colleges to get a thorough knowledge about the current research topic, with the knowledge acquired through the review materials. The researcher constructed an interview schedule covering all the objectives of the study. The primary data were collected directly from the respondent. The investigator conducted a face-to-face interview. Observation was made by the researcher. Apart from answers for the scheduled questions, other views and expressions of the respondents were also recorded very carefully. This information was very much useful for the research and the same were used in various places like interpretation of data and in summary of the conclusions. During the interview, privacy was maintained with the respondents to avoid the influence of neighbours on the interview. The secondary data were also collected and used in the study.

PRETEST

The schedule prepared was checked and the same was pretested by administering the questions with some (10 members) pregnant women. After the pretest, the researcher got an idea and some changes such as commission and omission of few questions and changing the patterns of questions were made. Without any ambiguity, the interview schedule was administered to collect first-hand information on the current topics.

ANALYSIS OF DATA

After the data collection, each schedule was checked for any shortcomings. The information was coded in numerical and entered into a master chart. From the master chart, the tables were formulated. Percentages were calculated for each category. The tables were interpreted in a scientific manner using the primary and secondary data.

SOCIAL BACKGROUND OF THE PREGNANT WOMEN

The social background plays a very important role in shaping a person's basic attitudes, values, health behaviour and health practices. In this chapter, an attempt has been made to bring out certain salient features and characteristics of the sample of pregnant women and

Table 14.1 Respondents Distributed by Selected Characteristics

Characteristic	*Number of Respondents*	*Total*
Age		
Less than 20	3	3
21–30	79	79
Above 30	18	18
Total (in %)	100	100
Literacy rate		
Literate	82	82
Illiterate	18	18
Total (in %)	100	100
Monthly income (in thousands)		
4,000–8,000	42	42
8,000–12,000	40	40
Above 12,000	18	18
Total (in %)	100	100
Types of family		
Nuclear family	71	71
Joint family	29	29
Total (in %)	100	100
Residential wealth status		
Own house	51	51
Rented house	49	49
Total (in %)	100	100
Classification of pregnant women		
Employed pregnant women	35	35
Unemployed pregnant Women	65	65
Total (in %)	100	100

their health status, socio-economic status and so on. With this background information, the researcher could explore some of the more complex dimensions of relation between the health condition and food pattern among the respondents—pregnant women.

Table 14.1 indicates that most of the respondents were between the age group of 21–30 years. Eighteen per cent of them fall into the age group above 30 years. They are forced to bear pregnancy after 30 years of age due to late marriage and health problems. Only 3 per cent belong to the age group less than 20 years. This is because of illiteracy and poverty. Eighty-two per cent of the respondents are literate. Remaining 18 per cent of the respondents are illiterate. Among the 82 per cent, majority of them have completed Higher Secondary School. Some of them have completed under graduation. Only a small number of respondents have studied post graduation. Eighteen per cent of the respondents could not obtain education due to poverty, lack of awareness, low income and more number of children in the family. Two per cent of the respondents' family is getting ₹4,000–8,000 as monthly income. Forty per cent are earning ₹ 8,000 to ₹12,000 as monthly income, whereas only 18 per cent respondent's family earn above ₹12,000 as monthly income.

Majority of the respondents experience nuclear families; most of the respondents' families have migrated from native rural area for education, employment, medical services and so on. Although 29 per cent of the sampled pregnant women were well satisfied staying in their parental home town, as many as 51 per cent of the respondents were having their own permanent residential accommodation in the city. Some of them from the above said percentage had sought loans with banks to own houses. Their repayment of loans, usually in instalments with interest has to be debited by the source company employer. Forty-nine per cent sampled pregnant women reside in rented house having financial problems, low income, family problems and so on. These classifications will increase and decrease on the population level based on the wealth status of the family. Some of the pregnant women were forced to take up employment due to commitment within the family.

As data framed in Table 14.2 show that 76 per cent of the sampled pregnant women are happy as they meet their anticipation, 16 per cent convinced themselves. Only 8 per cent of them who were unhappy resulted in third level (abortion) due to personal reasons

Table 14.2 Respondents Distributed Under Health of Pregnant Women and their Emotion and Anticipation Level, Health Condition

Characteristics	*Number of Respondents*	*Total*
Emotion and anticipation		
Happy	76	76
Accepting and convinced	16	16
Abortion	8	8
Total (in %)	100	100
Health condition		
Healthy	26	26
Weak	74	74
Total (in %)	100	100
Age for women to bear pregnancy		
Less than 20	1	1
21–30	98	98
Above 30	1	1
Total (in %)	100	100
Meals intaking intervals		
1 time	–	–
2 times	12	12
3 times	78	78
More than 3 times	10	10
Total(in %)	100	100
Hospitals preferred by samples for taking treatment		
Government hospital	87	87
Private hospital	13	13
Total (in %)	100	100

such as family problem, poverty, divorce and financial expenses on the family.

Seventy-four per cent of the sampled pregnant women felt the level of health condition of pregnant women today is considered too weak. This condition is due to general reasons such as low nutrients of food grains, processed medicines, environmental problems, low income, etc. Remaining 26 per cent of the respondents say that today's pregnant women are healthy due to awareness of health, health education, higher income and hygienic aspects. Ninety-eight per cent of the respondents say that between the age group of 21–30 years is the appropriate age for a woman to become pregnant. People who are all in the category of the age group of 21–30 years will be having adequate physical and mental soundness to bear and deliver a child. One per cent of the sampled pregnant women suggest that above 30 years of age will be the appropriate age for a woman to become pregnant. One per cent of the respondents say that the age group of below 20 years is the suitable age for a woman to bear a child.

Seventy-eight per cent of the pregnant women take meals three times a day. A small percentage of the sample take meals two times a day only in the morning and night with less vegetables and fruits. This situation continues due to low income, poverty, unemployment and carelessness, whereas 10 per cent take meals more than three times a day. The sampled pregnant women undergo some kind of medical treatment during their pregnancy depending upon their economic condition. Some seek government hospitals and some prefer private hospitals as per their paying capacity.

Eighty-seven per cent of the respondents undergo medical treatment in a government hospital. Thirteen per cent of the pregnant women undergo medical treatment in private hospitals due to high income, seeking better service and treatment with better scientific equipments that are easy to use.

Data, which are presented in Table 14.3, show that 68 per cent of the sampled pregnant women had anaemia. Seven per cent of the sample had low and high blood sugar. Seven per cent of the samples had jaundice. These pregnant women experienced weight loss and further, weight gain was experienced by 4 per cent of the sampled pregnant women. Only 8 per cent of the samples did not face any of those unhealthy consequences. People who belonged to the category of 8 per cent were taking rich nutritional food, whereas the remaining categories of people did not take nutritional food at proper time. The data presented in the table show that 63 per cent of the respondents advised that doing household works would be the best exercise during pregnancy period. Thirty-seven per cent of the respondents said that walking would be the best exercise for a pregnant woman to deliver a child in normal delivery. The majority seventy-one per cent of the respondents reported that they had strong

Table 14.3 Belief Patterns among the Respondents about the Effect of Reading Habit on the Growth of Intellectual Level of the Baby and the Mother.

Characteristics	*Number of Respondents*	*Total*
Unhealthy consequences		
Blood sugar	12	12
High blood pressure	7	7
Anaemia	60	60
Jaundice	6	6
Weight gain and loss	7	7
None of the above	8	8
Total (in %)	100	100
Types of exercise		
Household works	63	63
Walking	37	37
Total (in %)	100	100
Belief in reading habit of mothers and intellectual level of babies (% grade)		
Less	8	8
Average	21	21
Majority	71	71
Total (in %)	100	100

belief in the beneficial effect of reading habit of pregnant women on the growth of intellectual level of baby. An average level of 21 per cent had a medium level of belief. Less per cent (8) of the respondents had low level of belief.

An average of the sampled pregnant women who are educated in all hygienic aspects tend to use toilets in a hygienic and clean manner. As per data classified in the table, the researcher finds 51 per cent of the pregnant women use own toilet. Twenty-seven per cent of them use common toilets residing in line homes and have very less awareness of hygienic and health conditions. A certain per cent, that is less than 22 per cent, use corporation toilet or pay-and-use toilet provided by the Government Municipality where hygienic conditions are very less compared with the others. An average number of respondents are very eager to know the sex of the child during pregnancy itself. However, the Constitution Act does not permit it. Sixty-one per cent

Table 14.4 Impact of Mother's Mental Health on the Child Behaviour

S.No	*Behaviour Level*	*Number of Respondents*	*Total (%)*
1	Low behaviour level	3	3
2	Medium behaviour level	2	2
3	High behaviour level	95	95
	Total	**100**	**100**

of pregnant women prefer male child while remaining 49 per cent are satisfied with female child.

The data presented in the Table 14.4 show that most of the respondents (95 per cent) are advised to be in a good mental state (p atience), as they should not to be tensed by work or family stress, which might have an impact on the child's behaviour levels. This will lead to comfort and happiness in the family. Ninety-five per cent of the respondents have high belief on the above statements. Two per cent of the respondents believe to some extent. The remaining 3 per cent of the respondents believe in low behaviour level due to illiteracy and lack of awareness.

The data in Table 14.5 show that the respondents express that mothers' education will have a direct impact on their children's nutrition. An educated mother will take care of the child's intake nutritionally. A majority (61 per cent) of the respondents accepted their educational level will impact greatly on the child's nutrition intake. Thirty-five per cent of the respondents depended on aged persons in the family regarding the intake of child nutrition biologically. The least number (4 per cent) of respondents are illiterate and have no awareness on the above-said relationship or the importance behind it.

Table 14.5 Level of Believeness among the Respondents on the Relationship of Mother's Education and Child's Malnutrition

S.No	*Level of Believeness (in %)*	*Number of Respondents*	*Total (%)*
1	Low	4	4
2	Average	35	35
3	Majority	61	61
	Total	100	100

CONCLUSION

The present study covers the respondents in the age group between 20 and 30 years. The outcome of the study clearly explains that majority of the respondents (pregnant women) belonged to the age group of 21–30 years, and they considered the age between 21 and 30 years is suitable for women to bear pregnancy and childbirth because the age group of a woman has an adequate strength both physically and mentally to bear and deliver a child.

The majority of the respondents in this study reside in their own houses. The small size of the sampled pregnant women resides in rental houses. The researcher found that most of the respondents who are living as a nuclear family and few per cent of the respondents who are living as joint family and have the native background shifted from rural areas. The respondents wanted to reside with their mothers' house where they grow up till delivery. It helps the respondents to have access to health care knowledge from their mothers, relax from serious work burdens, seek health services near to their parents' residence and trained to take care of their child after delivery.

The study found that most of the respondents (pregnant women) confirmed their pregnancy through Home Pregnancy Test by experienced symptoms, such as tender, swollen breasts, fatigue, implantation bleeding, nausea or vomiting. A small portion of the respondents have undergone Medical Pregnancy Test immediately to confirm their pregnancy.

The researcher found that 70 per cent of the respondents (pregnant women) were aware about their health condition, the value of nutritional food and started to concentrate on their health and hygiene of the environment around them. The remaining 30 per cent were not aware of their health condition, and they did not concentrate on their health and hygiene. Though they were aware of their health condition, they were not in a position to take any efforts for improvement due to poverty, illiteracy and low income and so on.

A pregnant woman has emotional feelings after the conformation of her pregnancy. The emotional feelings of happiness are categorized into happy, accepting and convinced to abortion. Majority of the respondents (pregnant women) feel happy about their pregnancy. Only 2 per cent of respondents opt for abortion due to poverty or already having more number of children.

In this study, the pregnant women have different opinions about the health condition of today's pregnant women. The pregnant women have opined that today's pregnant women's health has become very poor. The researcher found that the health condition of pregnant women today is too weak compared with that of pregnant women in olden days. This continued due to intake of food grains, vegetables and fruits, which are exposed to chemicals, fertilizers and pesticides for quick productivity, which has low content of nutritional power in it.

The respondents (pregnant women) who belong to the age group between 21 and 30 years have experienced pregnancy for the very first time. The researcher found that the large portion of the pregnant women get all kinds of support from their family members. Three-fourth of the husbands of the respondents say that they meet all kinds of help for them in household works such as cooking, washing, cleaning the house and giving psychological support with abundant love and affection.

The study brought out the fact that the large number of pregnant women intake three times of meals a day with fruits, vegetables and dairy products. They intake nutritional food, which accumulates rich protein, energy, carbohydrate, fat, calcium, iron and fibre in their body. Among the respondents, a huge number of pregnant women belonged to the weight of 40–50 kg. A small portion of the respondents belonged to the weight category of 50–60 kg. The respondents who belong to the weight category of below 40 kg are considered weak/malnourished. Weight of the pregnant women varies from one another on monthly basis and depends on the growth of the child in them.

The researcher found the fact that the pregnant women undergo medical treatment from government and private hospitals. The pregnant women undergo treatment at government hospital, and a meagre number of pregnant women undergo treatment at private hospitals for monthly check-up and medical tests periodically. These pregnant women undergo various tests such as blood pressure level, blood sugar level, HIV test, urinary test, scanning and weight on monthly basis. Among the respondents, a large number of pregnant women face unhealthy consequences during pregnancy.

The respondents get benefited by PHC headed by ICTC to get all kinds of medicines and vaccination at respective time frames. The PHC centres play a vital role in the health and maintenance of pregnant women and concerned on the child's growth and deficiency levels also. The pregnant women are provided healthy food which contains all kinds of vitamins, proteins, fibres, carbohydrate and so on. They get health education through Health Induction Programme organized by PHCs. The 'Health Induction Programme' educate these pregnant women about how to lead their life in a healthy and hygienic environment, how to protect child and themselves from spreading diseases such as cholera, malaria and flu. Newly formulated vaccination is injected to pregnant women to avoid contracting communicable diseases. The respondents are subject to vaccination under tetanus toxoid twice during pregnancy with different intervals to avoid getting diseases.

It is important to note that ICTC does not stop providing vaccination and medicines. It also helps the pregnant women to get financial support from the government-aided organization under welfare scheme to pregnant women, as every pregnant woman will be provided ₹ 6,000 and ₹ 7,500.

In the present study, the pregnant women opined that working during pregnancy will be a good exercise for the pregnant women for easy delivery of child. They were advised house exercise. Some of the respondents were advised walking as a good exercise for them to experience easy delivery and to avoid caesarean section, which most of them do not prefer.

The respondents expressed that mother's education has a close relationship with their children's nutrition. An educated mother will take care of the child's intake nutritionally. A majority of the respondents accept that educational level will greatly impact on the child's nutrition intake. An average of them depended on aged persons in the family regarding the intake of child nutrition biologically. Four per cent of the respondents who are illiterate have no awareness on the above said relationship or the importance behind it.

The respondents expressed that their health can become better by improving some areas such as utilizing Primary Health Care services, taking nutritive food, creating awareness, involvement of government and non-government organizations in providing medical treatment with advanced equipments and medicines, implementing new welfare schemes in improving health status of pregnant women.

Every woman has the right to health especially during pregnancy and childbirth. Health care providers should be technically competent and should treat women with respect. Quality health care enables women to make informed decisions about their health by offering information and counselling. It should be easy for women who need maternal care to reach the health facility.

REFERENCES

Florez, C.E. and D.P. Hogan, 1990, 'Women's Status and Infant Mortality in Rural Colombia', *Social Biology*, 37(3–4): 188–203.

Kulkarni, S., S. Ahani and S. Seetharam, 1996, 'Maternal Mortality Bellary (1998-1992)', *Journal of Obstetrics and Gynaecology of India*, 46: 492.

Kwalombota, M., 2002, 'The Effect of Pregnancy in HIV-Infected Women', *AIDS Care*, 14(3): 431–33.

Lawoyin, T.O. and U. Larsen, 2002, 'Male Sexual Behaviour During Wife's Pregnancy and Postpartum Abstinence Period in Oyo State, Nigeria', *Journal of Biosocial Science*, 34(1): 51–63.

Mercer, Alex, Nowsher Uddin, Nafisa Lira Huq, Fariha Haseen, Mobarak Hossain Khan and Charles P. Larson, 2006, 'Validating Neonatal Mortality and use of NGO Reproductive Health Outreach Services in Rural Bangladesh', *Studies in Family Planning*, 37(2): 111–22.

Naik, Poonam, 2011, 'Safe Motherhood', *Health Journal*, 89(1): 33–5.

Sravani, V.L., 2011, 'OTC Drugs to be Avoided in Pregnancy', *Health Journal*, 89(6): 17–9.

Sujatha, V., 2003, *Health by the People: Sociology of Medical Lore*. Jaipur and New Delhi: Rawat Publications, pp. 15, 21–27, 38.

The Hindu, 2011, Online edition of India's National Newspaper, Sunday, 5 June.

UNDP, 1998, 'Nepal Human Development Report', studied and published by Nepal South Asia Centre and submitted the report to UNDP, Kathmandu, Nepal, pp. 56–74.

UNFPA, 2002, 'HIV Prevention among Pregnant Women and Newborns'. In *HIV/AIDS Prevention Guidance for Reproductive Health Professionals in Developing–Country Settings*, New York: Population Council, pp. 38–48.

UNICEF, 2006, 'Situation of Children and Women in Nepal: A Situation Analysis', published by United Nations Children's Fund, Nepal Country Office, UN House, Kathmandu, Nepal, p. 3.

Velkoff, V.A. and A. Adlakha, 1998, 'Women's Health in India', *Women's of the World*, published by International Programs Centre, U.S. Census Bureau, the Official Statistics™. 10 December 1998, WID/98–3.

World Health Organization (WHO), 2001, 'Men, Aging and Health', published by WHO, Geneva, 01WHO/NMH/ NPH 01.2, p. 10.

Index